TRAIN LIKE A FIGHTER

TRAIN LIKE A FIGHTER

BY CAT ZINGANO

ALPHA

CONTENTS

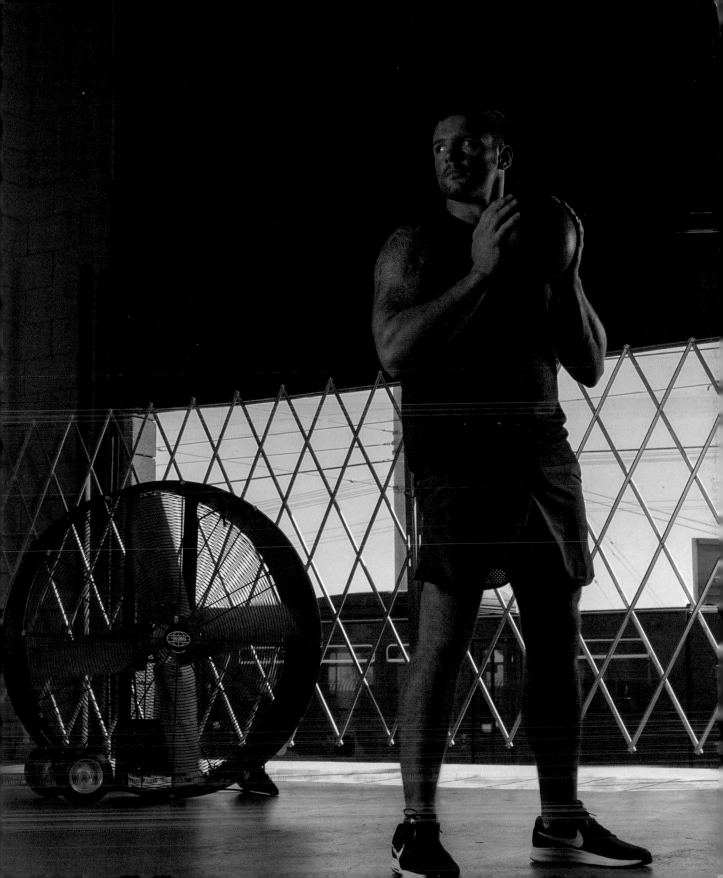

FOREWORD

Like all competitive athletes, martial artists travel roads that demand vision, sacrifice, and commitment on a daily basis. During this journey, we're constantly reminded that the destination isn't the goal—the adventure we embark on is. I've been fortunate to have been on a journey with my friend Cat Zingano for the last six years. I was introduced to Cat by one of her MMA coaches. Our first training session together told me all I needed to know about her. Cat's work ethic is unparalleled, and her attempt to exhaust herself in every aspect of training showed me her mental fortitude.

What's truly impressive about Cat is her thirst for knowledge, wanting to understand the *why* and *how*, and her level of coachability was a game-changer for me! I could tell during that first training session that she was the type of person who would push you to earn her trust. She wasn't going to cut me any slack based on any other MMA fighter I had ever worked with. She wanted to know that whomever was in charge of her physical preparation for competition truly cared about her and wasn't just providing a one-size-fits-all training model. She was cautious in conversation yet stubborn in debate. I knew from personal experience with other athletes that if I could become one of her coaches that this was going to be as much of a learning journey for me as it was her—and I was right!

During our time together, I've seen her climb the mountain and fight for the UFC bantamweight title as well as overcome obstacles that would make most people quit. She's been tested professionally and personally time and time again— and her resilience won out time and time again, helping her become stronger and stronger. How Cat approaches training has become a metaphor for how she handles difficult things in her life: head-on and not looking back.

In fact, Cat's work ethic has been the beacon during dark and difficult times. This book is an insight into the methods that have helped her compete on the biggest stage in the world of MMA—fighting in the UFC as the number one contender in the bantamweight division—but more importantly, these are the daily methods she has used to overcome the trials and tribulations of life to give her the resolve of a champion! I've been fortunate to watch Cat go through these exact exercises and workouts. Her intensity, focus, and intent while training are what separate her from all other MMA fighters. Use this book as a guide for better health and performance, but more importantly, see this book as a road map to take on anything life might throw your way!

I can honestly say that being one of Cat's coaches has helped me become a better coach, but I've also gained a great friend during this journey together! So please join me on this journey to a new you—inside and out—with Cat Zingano to guide us!

Loren Landow
strength and conditioning coach
and owner of Landow Performance

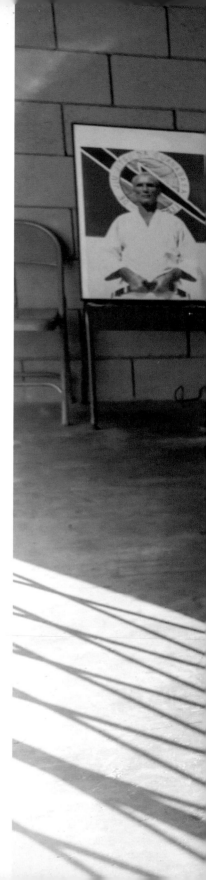

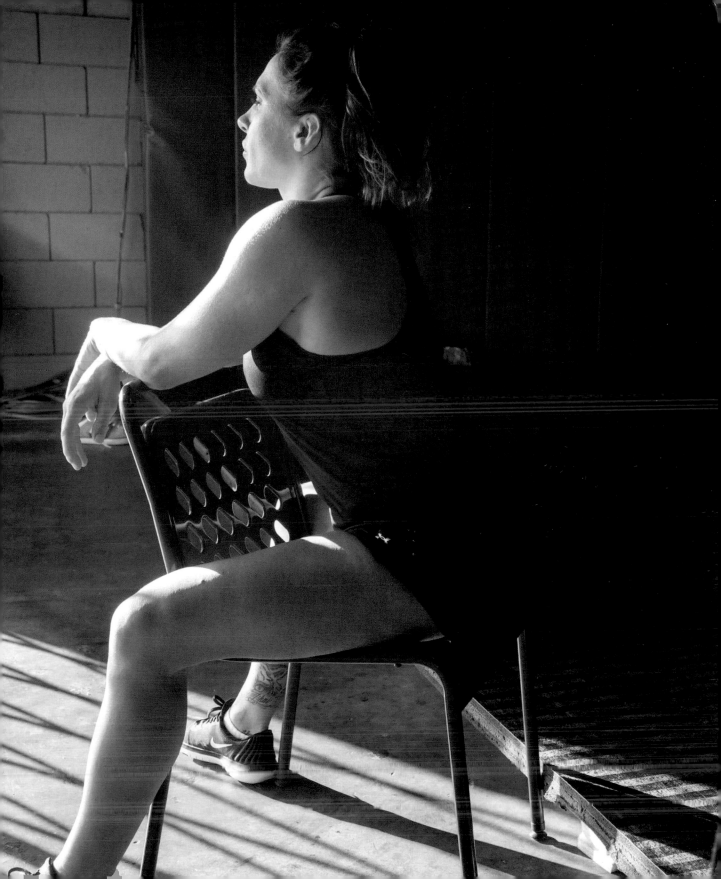

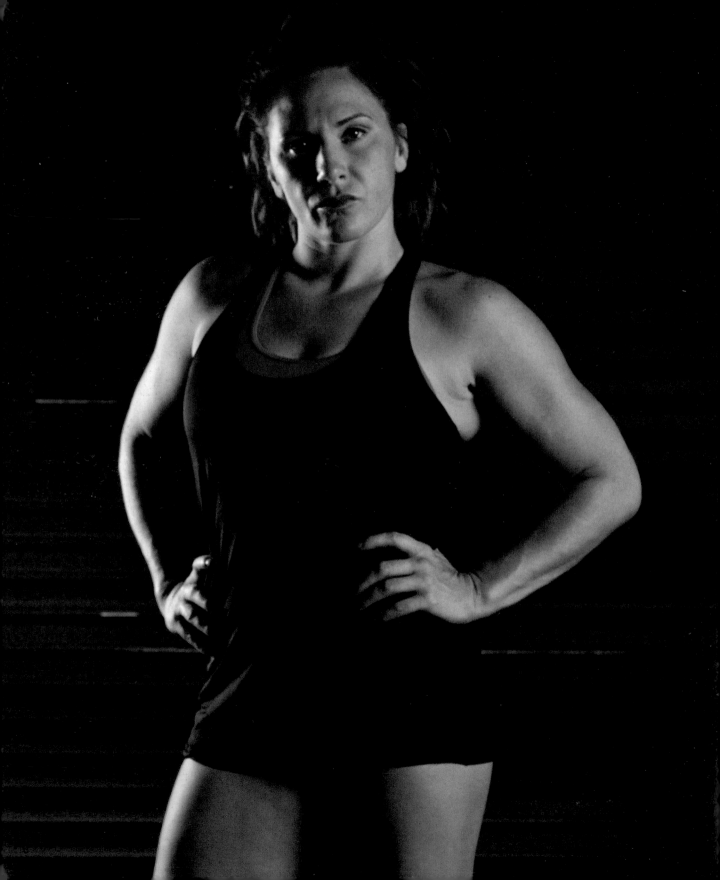

INTRODUCTION

My athletic and combative sports journey started when I was very young. I always found peace and enjoyment in playing, competing, and seeing results at the end of setting goals. I'll admit, I was troubled growing up, where sports and staying active were my most effective therapy. When I was in a gym or out on a field, my mind was right and I felt calm— the quiet from my troubles came from being physical. On a team, being coached and setting goals kept me company and always made me feel supported and important, learning to optimize my results by putting myself and my training first. I figured out that I need to move, I realized I need to be able to hold myself accountable, and I still know that keeping things changing is important for keeping my attention.

I participated in many sports and got very good at them. Finding combative sports and expressive motions eventually became my identity. There was always more to do, and there were always new goals to set. The personal accomplishment that came with learning how to physically protect yourself and your loved ones practically was extremely attractive to me. And while I was learning and working toward an understanding of these possibilities and methods, I found a way of living. I would look down and see my body. I liked what I looked like, but more so, I loved what I could do. It wasn't about the scale (although I am in a weight-class-sensitive sport); it was about showing myself what I could do, how strong I could be, and how much health could be earned.

In 2006, I had my wonderful baby boy, Brayden Matthew. Wanting to give him a healthy mom and comfortable life in mind, I started working out on my off hours from school. I had to balance being a new mom, taking classes as a full-time student studying to become an ASL (American Sign Language) interpreter, and working to pay the bills. The gym was tedious. I hated paying a monthly fee for something so boring and with so little evidence of results. I needed to play—just like when I was a kid.

I tried to go to jazzercise, I picked up dance classes, and I spent time on gym equipment— only to feel completely annoyed. Although these workouts had their place in my life at one point, I needed more now. I was a former athlete, a new single mom, a full-time student—and I needed a stronger outlet than mundane workouts.

I then found Brazilian jiu-jitsu, wanted to challenge myself, and started pretty quickly toward wanting to compete in MMA. I remember seeing the strong, confident gait of mixed martial artists, and I wanted to do what they do, but I needed to know what they knew. It was beautiful to me—the whole package.

I started in mixed martial arts because I found a way to move my body in a self-expressive movement, where I barely noticed working out because I was chasing objectives: performance and outlet. While focusing on and setting my goals in competition, the weight started to fall off, my body started to tighten, I became more loose and flexible, and, most importantly, I liked myself. I lost the baby weight, and I got stronger—mentally and physically— along the way. Every day, I trained to improve—and I did because I went there exactly for that reason.

We all crave challenges and to be able to openly express ourselves creatively. Many people use motion and movement as a physical outlet. Especially me. My journey has been learning most things in life the hard way. And I'm grateful for the lessons. I've learned that fear defines your limits; pushing your limits and continuing to move through them benefits your confidence and self-esteem from the inside out.

Although the exercises in this book are hard at times, getting through them will grow your level of self-worth and show you what you can create. This book is about finding yourself through movement and learning to fight, stretch, strengthen, and express yourself with physical activity.

Cat Zingano

ABOUT THE MODELS

If you want to look like a fighter, then you need to learn from those who fight for a living. The publisher wishes to thank these athletes for showing how to perform the exercises in this book.

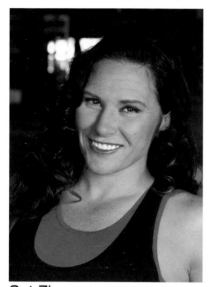

Cat Zingano
Winona, Minnesota

Cat grew up in Boulder, Colorado, where she started wrestling in middle school. She then wrestled in high school and college, winning two national titles and twice being named an all-American. Soon after experiencing Brazilian jiu-jitsu for the first time in 2007, she won the world championship in Los Angeles and the Rio de Janiero state championship in Brazil. After those wins, she competed in her first MMA fight, which eventually led to her becoming a top contender in the UFC.

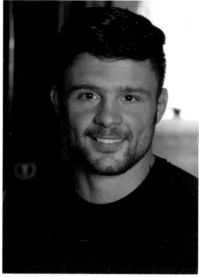

Tarsis Humphreys
São Paulo, Brazil

Tarsis is a professional Brazilian jiu-jitsu competitor in the black belt division. In 2009, he won the first World Professional Jiu Jitsu Cup (now the Abu Dhabi World Pro) in his weight class and in the open weight class. He's won several International Brazilian Jiu-Jitsu Federation (IBJJF) competitions: the world championship in 2010; the Pan American championship in 2006 (weight and open class); the European Open championship in 2010; and the Los Angeles BJJ pro championship in 2016.

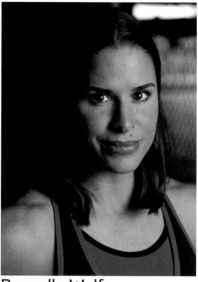

Danyelle Wolf
York, Pennsylvania

Danyelle never touched boxing gloves until 2008, but she's had a lot of success in the sport since, including making Team USA's Olympic boxing squad. She was the USA National Boxing Champion in 2013, 2014, and 2015; the Continental Champion in 2013 and 2015; the Ringside World Champion in 2012, 2013, and 2014; and the Golden Gloves National Champion in 2014. After also winning three Brazilian jiu-jitsu titles in 2016, she's preparing to transition to an MMA career.

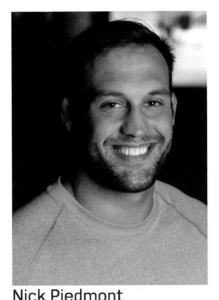

Nick Piedmont
Tucson, Arizona

Nick is an MMA competitor who fights in the featherweight division of Bellator MMA. Although he wrestled as a young child, he wanted to do more, so he started boxing and performing jiu-jitsu. He began his career on the Arizona circuit but moved to California to push himself personally and professionally. It was a decision that came after two losses but with an eagerness and a hunger for an opportunity to pursue his talents as a fighter—and he's making the most of that choice.

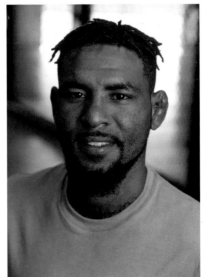

Darrion Caldwell
Rahway, New Jersey

Darrion is an MMA fighter who competes in the bantamweight division of Bellator MMA. As a high school wrestler, he won three state titles. He continued that success as a wrestler at North Carolina State, where he won a national title in 2009, defeating 2008 Dan Hodge Trophy winner Brent Metcalf in the finals, whom he also beat in 2008—the only blemish on Metcalf's record those seasons. He began fighting in MMA in 2012 and has steadily found success.

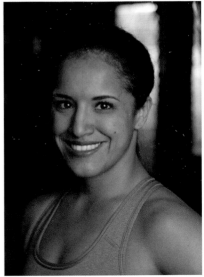

Paulina Granados
Ingleside, Texas

Paulina competes in MMA in the atomweight division in Combate Americas. Although she's had success as a Muay Thai fighter and in grappling, what she really enjoys about MMA is the boxing aspects. Despite her small stature, she prefers a stand-up fighting style that can bewilder her opponents. Even though she's been an athlete since she was four years old, she's found a home in MMA, where she can combine different techniques into one fight experience.

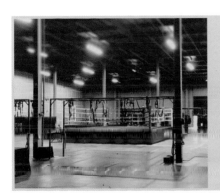

Alliance Training Center
Located in San Diego, the Alliance Training Center offers mixed martial arts and fitness training for up-and-coming athletes as well as seasoned MMA veterans. The facility also encourages people from all walks of life to reap the benefits of a healthy, active lifestyle in a family-first environment. Thanks to Eric Del Fierro and Brandon Vera for the opportunity to photograph this book at Alliance. And special thanks to Rolando Perez and the staff at Alliance for helping everyone away from home for the photo shoot feel like they're at home.

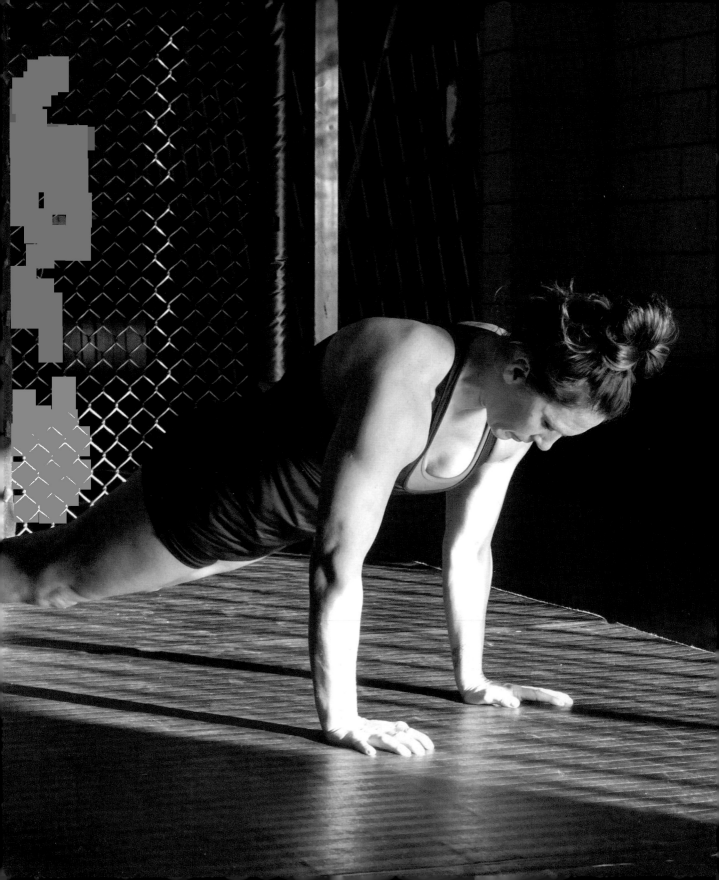

TRAINING BASICS

WHY TRAIN LIKE A FIGHTER?

Training like a fighter is more than exercise. It's a form of self-expression and a great physical outlet. But getting fit like an MMA fighter has benefits beyond looking ripped.

TO IMPROVE YOUR STRENGTH

Performing the cardiovascular, aerobic, and bodyweight exercises in this book can increase your heart rate; boost your endorphins; burn fat and maintain muscle; and help develop and maintain your muscle mass. Being stronger and more dynamic means more stamina, energy, and confidence for taking on any task. Don't be surprised if you find yourself subconsciously applying your fighter training regimen and work ethic to other aspects of your life.

TO IMPROVE YOUR POWER

Better power means more efficient strength and speed by collectively focusing on explosiveness, form, and agility. Having increased power comes from a strong foundation of balance and symmetry. That's why exercises in this book either work your body symmetrically or you perform reps independently on both sides of your body—one after the other. These exercises also test your physical and mental perseverance by constantly redefining your limits, helping to enhance your drive, flexibility, and endurance.

TO IMPROVE YOUR STABILITY

When you've dialed in your strength and power, you're also going to have more stability. This is because maintaining your position and actively engaging different body parts automatically demand that you focus on balance, which depends on a stronger lower body and base. The exercises in this book can help you gain that improved balance as well as help you develop better cardio and a skill set that allows you to confidently take on things you might have thought were impossible.

> "Fighter training is a way to help you match your inside to your outside— with **strength, poise,** and **confidence.**"

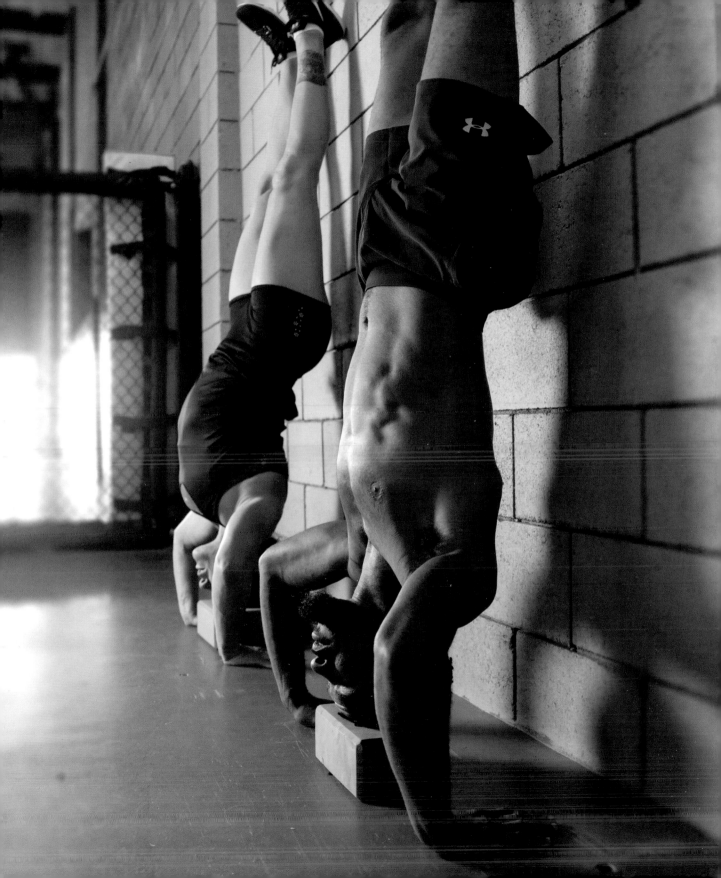

COMMON FIGHTER MOVES

Many exercises in this book include variations on basic MMA fighting moves. Knowing how to perform the original moves with proper form and stances can help you with your productivity, workout flow, and body movement goals.

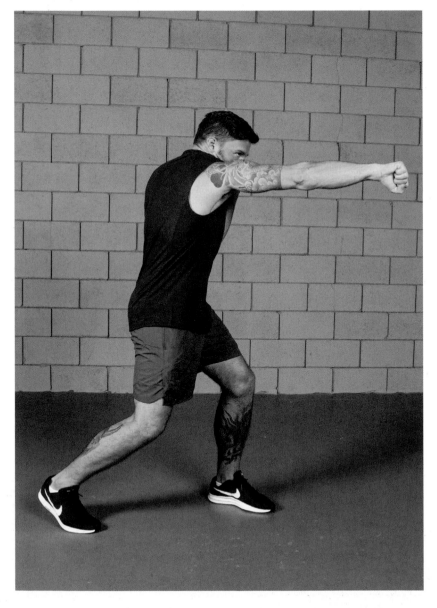

Jabs

1. Stagger your feet, placing the toe of your right foot about 18–25 inches behind the heel of your left foot, and slightly bend your knees.

2. Hold your balled hands at your cheekbones, with your knuckles toward your face.

3. Twist at your hips and quickly extend your right arm out at eye level, twisting your wrist so your thumb points down.

4. Lift only the heel of your back foot when throwing a jab, and keep your back straight rather than lean into the punch.

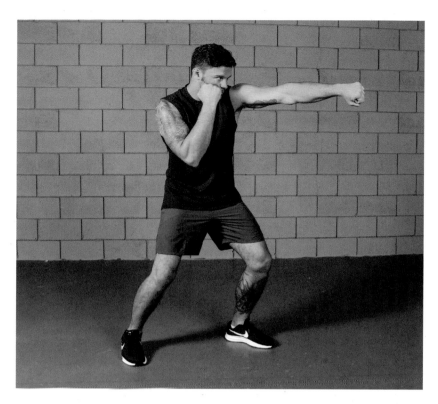

Crosses

1. Stagger your feet, placing your right foot about 18–25 inches behind your left foot, turning your right foot until it's perpendicular to your body and angling your left foot more toward your left side.

2. Keep your knees slightly bent, and keep your feet flat on the ground as well as keep your back straight when punching.

3. Hold your balled hands at your cheekbones, with your knuckles toward your face.

4. Twist at your hips and quickly extend your left arm out at eye level, twisting your wrist so your thumb points down.

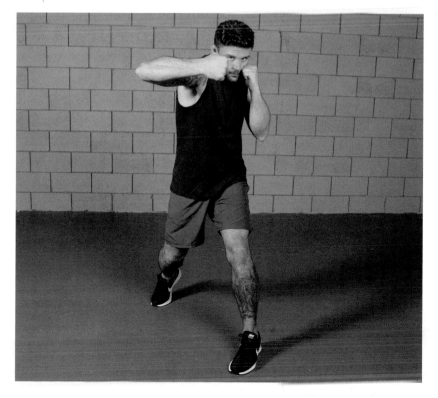

Hooks

1. Stagger your feet, placing your right foot about 18–25 inches behind your left foot, and slightly bend your knees.

2. Hold your balled hands at your cheekbones, with your knuckles toward your face.

3. Twist at your hips and quickly extend your right arm across your face at eye level, twisting your wrist so your thumb points up.

4. Lift only the heel of your back foot when throwing a jab, pivoting on your left foot, and keep your back straight rather than lean into the punch.

Elbows #1

1. Stagger your feet, placing your left foot about 18–25 inches behind your right foot, turning your left foot until it's perpendicular to your body and angling your right foot more toward your right side.

2. Keep your knees slightly bent, and step your right foot slightly forward as you swing your right elbow out or upward.

3. Use your left hand to protect the left side of your face or engage your left arm to help with momentum.

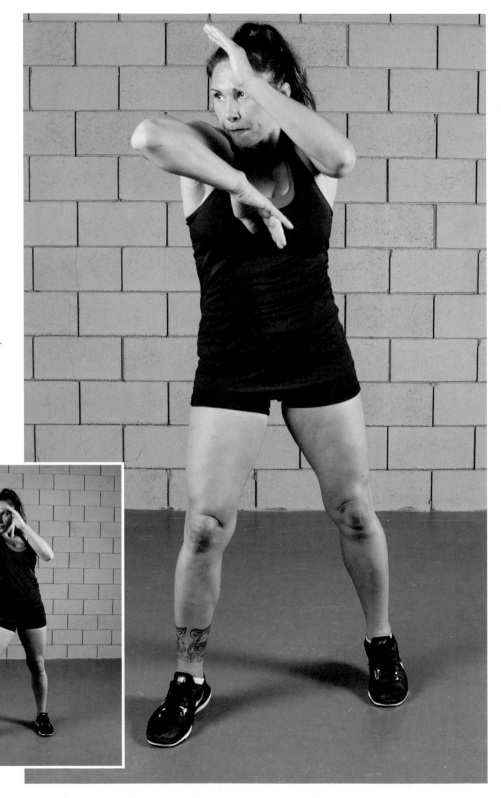

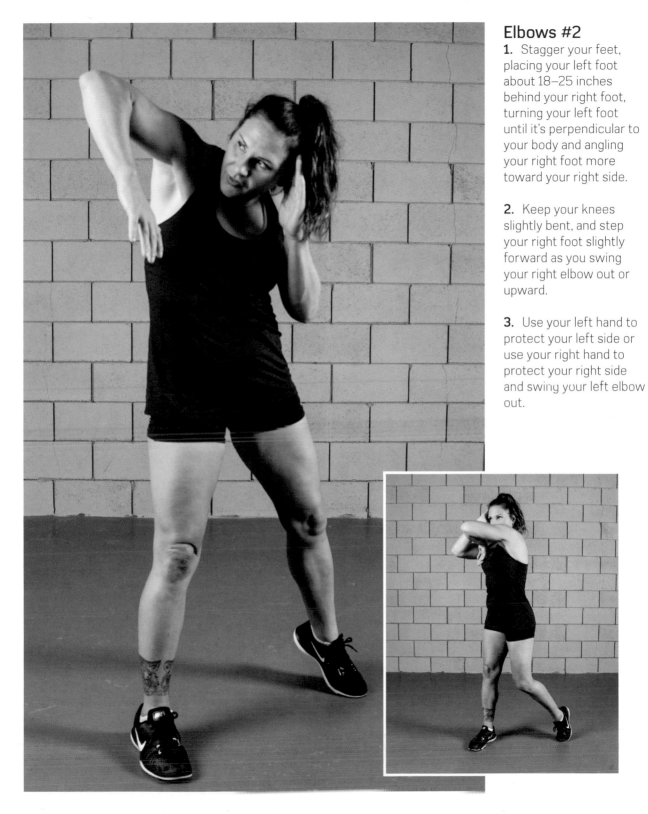

Elbows #2

1. Stagger your feet, placing your left foot about 18–25 inches behind your right foot, turning your left foot until it's perpendicular to your body and angling your right foot more toward your right side.

2. Keep your knees slightly bent, and step your right foot slightly forward as you swing your right elbow out or upward.

3. Use your left hand to protect your left side or use your right hand to protect your right side and swing your left elbow out.

Knees

1. Stagger your feet, placing your right foot about 18–25 inches behind your left foot, turning your left foot until it's perpendicular to your body and angling your right foot more toward your right side.

2. Keep your right leg straight, lifting just the heel of your right foot off the ground, and lift your right knee up toward your chest, swinging your left arm out to the side and bringing your right arm in front of your face for protection.

3. Alternatively, you can switch your initial leg placements and switch the other arm and leg movements.

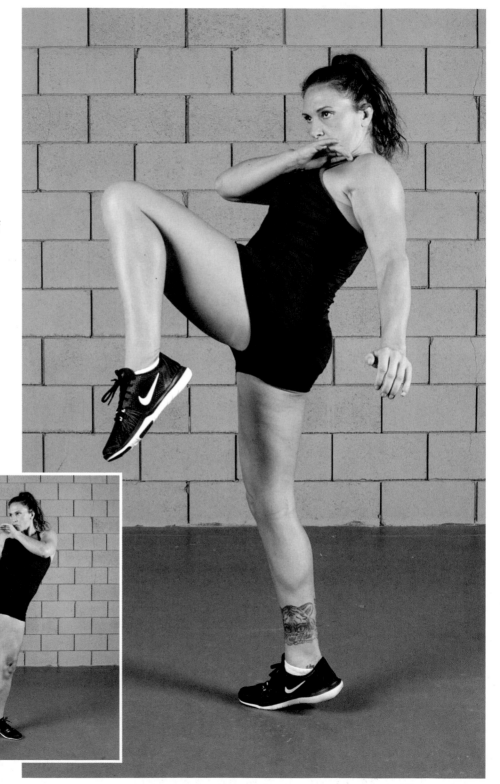

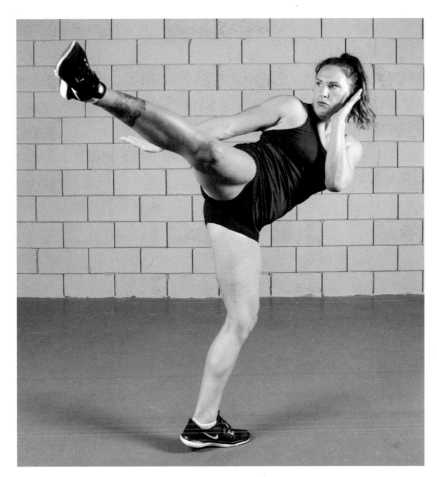

Kicks

1. Stagger your feet, placing your left foot about 18–25 inches behind your right foot, turning your right foot until it's perpendicular to your body and angling your left foot more toward your left side.

2. Slightly bend your left knee, then kick your right leg out in front of you, also keeping a slight bend in that knee.

3. Swing your right arm out to the side and bringing your left hand to the left side of your face for protection, twisting at your hips for momentum.

4. Allow only the heel of your left foot to come off the ground, pivoting on that foot.

5. Alternatively, you can switch your initial leg placements and switch the other arm and leg movements.

Using moves for warmups & cooldowns

These four drills are efficient ways to get your heart rate going and to warm up your joints. Use one or more to help energize your muscles.

Although the moves in these drills are meant to be done with speed and form in mind, if you do them slowly, they're ideal for cooldowns and shakeouts.

DRILL 1

Perform these moves in order or in reverse—doing as many of each as you desire.

Crosses ▶ Kicks ▶ Knees ▶ Elbows #1 ▶ Jabs

DRILL 3

Perform these moves in order or in reverse—doing as many of each as you desire.

Knees ▶ Jabs ▶ Elbows #2 ▶ Hooks ▶ Kicks

DRILL 2

Perform these moves in order or in reverse—doing as many of each as you desire.

Hooks ▶ Knees ▶ Elbows #2 ▶ Kicks ▶ Crosses

DRILL 4

Perform these moves in order or in reverse—doing as many of each as you desire.

Kicks ▶ Crosses ▶ Knees ▶ Jabs ▶ Elbows #1

EQUIPMENT

Some exercises in this book require equipment to help you perform workouts, challenge different muscles, and produce maximum results for your goals. Your gym should have most of this equipment.

HAND WRAPS
Wraps can offer some support and security when training intensely, allowing you to focus on your form rather than worrying about injuring your hands.

DUMBBELLS
Use dumbbells that feel comfortable in your hands. Start with lighter weights, then incrementally use heavier ones as you begin to feel more comfortable.

STEP PLATFORM
Some exercises in this book use this for elevating your body off the ground or to support your upper body. Most also have the ability to change height.

KETTLEBELLS

Kettlebells are heavy cast iron or cast steel weights. Use light ones that feel comfortable in your hands before working your way up to heavier ones.

PLYOMETRIC BOX

A plyo box comes in wood, foam, and steel as well as different heights. Use one that supports your weight and capabilities, especially after repeated use.

HEAVY BAG

Boxing bags go by many different names, including heavy bag and punching bag. Use one that has some give but also offers some resistance.

SOCCER BALL

Find a soccer ball that can handle being stepped on often. You might also use a soccer ball to help ease you into using a medicine ball for throwing exercises.

YOGA MAT

Training often requires a lot of time on the ground. Using a yoga mat means a more comfortable surface for your body and better traction for your feet.

MEDICINE BALLS

Medicine balls usually come in a wide range of weights and sizes, so find one that pushes you toward using a heavier one as you build up your strength.

WEIGHT PLATE

Barbell weights— or plates—come in different weights and sizes. Start with one that has light resistance and work up to a heavier one.

NUTRITION WHEN TRAINING

If you're training to look like an MMA fighter, then you need to develop an MMA fighter's dietary habits. If some of these tips are new to you, pick one to try every day for two weeks. If they work, keep them. If they don't, try something else.

HABITS TO BUILD

▶ **Eat slowly.** Your body digests food slowly, so if you also eat your food more slowly, you're better able to know when you're full.

▶ **Drink more water.** This can help you regulate your body temperature as well as keep your joints lubricated before, during, and after exercising.

▶ **Create a daily meal plan.** Knowing when you're going to eat and how often can help you plan your exercise times as well as ensure you eat enough.

▶ **Eat more whole food sources.** Eating fewer processed foods and more low-calorie foods (and high in carbs) can help with weight loss.

▶ **Eat more lean protein.** Aid recovery and keep your muscle mass lean by eating more protein.

▶ **Eat more fruits and vegetables.** You'll get more needed fiber, vitamins, and minerals if you eat a wide variety of fruits and vegetables.

▶ **Eat a variety of foods.** Rotate the foods you like so you're getting a wide range of different nutrients and don't get bored with what you eat.

▶ **Eat healthy fats.** Eating healthy fats can help you lose body fat even during your everyday activities.

▶ **Eat in moderation (but don't feel guilty).** No one's perfect—just strive for less cheating.

Eating before and after training

This book can't tell you exactly what to eat each day because everyone has different needs, but these suggestions offer some basic guidelines for what you can eat before and after training to ensure you have the best experience possible without hurting your goals.

Keep in mind that not everyone reacts to certain foods in the same way. If you know a food might cause you problems—or you just don't like it—look for something similar to replace it with. The key to staying focused on your diet goals is to develop and maintain a routine.

BEFORE TRAINING

Start with this plan and modify it as needed.

TRAINING MEALS
▶ Lean protein: 2 palm-sized servings for men and 1 palm-sized serving for women
▶ Vegetables: 2 fist-sized servings for men and 1.5 fist-sized servings for women
▶ Carbs for each meal: 2 cupped-hands-size servings for men and 1.5 cupped-hands-size servings for women
▶ Healthy fats for each meal: 2 thumb-sized servings for men and 1 thumb-sized servings for women

AFTER TRAINING

Plan your meals so you're eating about an hour after exercising. This way, you'll gain muscle and mass—but stay focused on balance.

POST-WORKOUT MEALS
▶ Lean protein to help rebuild muscle damage and to maintain your energy level
▶ Vegetables high in vitamins and minerals to help gain back those lost during exercise
▶ Carbs to help level out your blood glucose as well as replenish lost muscle glucose stores
▶ Healthy fats—in moderation—to help you better digest other foods

What about supplements?

Complementing your exercise and diet with some all-natural supplements—additions to your meals and not strictly as replacements for them—can help with workout recovery. Talk with a nutrititionist or a dietician about adding these to your diet.

▶ **Green tea:** Drinking this can improve your stamina and boost your metabolism, which increases your endurance, allowing you to exercise longer. It's also conducive for brain health, and its antioxident properties aid in burning fat and helping you avoid autoimmune diseases.

▶ **Protein shakes:** Enjoying a protein-rich shake after a workout helps with muscle health and repair as well as delivers essential nutrients to depleted organs and muscles. Occasionally replacing meals with a protein shake can help you lose weight while still maintaining a healthy diet while also burning more calories than you consume.

▶ **Multivitamins:** Taking these with food in the morning, depending on your workout time, is highly recommended. It's often difficult to get proper and efficient nutrients from our food alone. You can take fish oil capsules for omega-3 fatty acids; probiotics for digestive health; and magnesium and vitamin D for a variety of body functions. It's best, though, to not take any of these right before or after a workout.

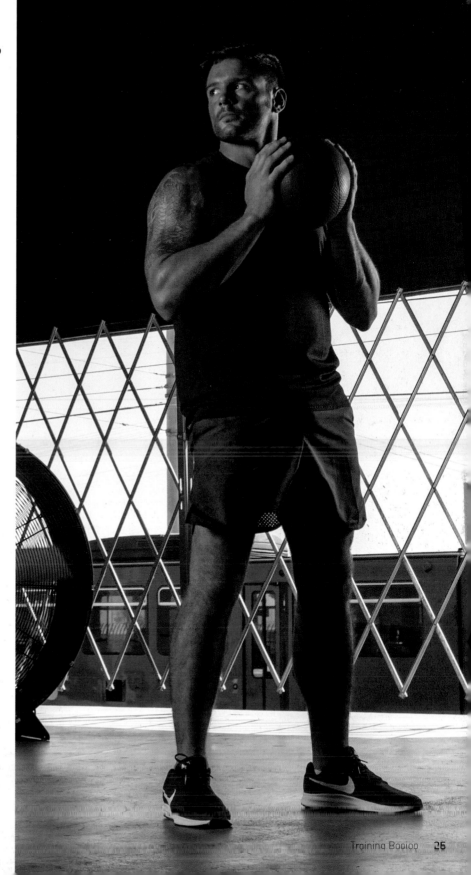

USING THIS BOOK

Training intelligently is more useful than training hard. This book offers three different ways—which when done in combination can contribute to each other—for helping you reach your physical and fitness goals.

EXERCISES

From building defined muscles in your arms to strengthening your legs and tightening your abs, the 60 exercises in this book target three key areas—upper body, core, and lower body— as well as offer several full-body experiences.

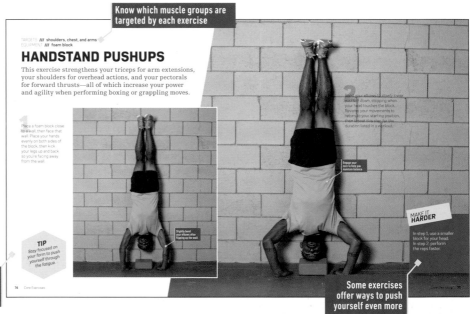

Know which muscle groups are targeted by each exercise

TARGETS /// shoulders, chest, and arms
EQUIPMENT /// foam block

HANDSTAND PUSHUPS

This exercise strengthens your triceps for arm extensions, your shoulders for overhead actions, and your pectorals for forward thrusts—all of which increase your power and agility when performing boxing or grappling moves.

Place a foam block close to a wall, then face that wall. Place your hands evenly on both sides of the block, then kick your legs up and back so you're facing away from the wall.

Bend your elbows to slowly lower yourself down, stopping when your head touches the block. Reverse your movements to return to your starting position, then repeat this step for the duration listed in a workout.

Engage your core to help you maintain balance.

Slightly bend your elbows after flipping up the wall.

MAKE IT HARDER

In step 1, use a smaller block for your head. In step 2, perform the reps faster.

TIP
Stay focused on your form to push yourself through the fatigue.

74   Core Exercises

Tips provide helpful advice on proper form and movement

Some exercises offer ways to push yourself even more

WORKOUTS

Filled with exercises presented in circuits, the 20 workouts can help you build endurance, increase muscle mass, and develop speed, agility, and flexibility— all within one routine.

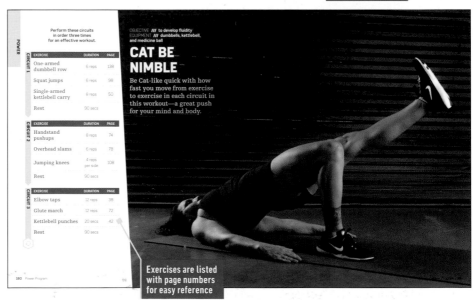

POWER

Perform these circuits in order three times for an effective workout.

OBJECTIVE /// to develop fluidity
EQUIPMENT /// dumbbells, kettlebell, and medicine ball

CAT BE NIMBLE

Be Cat-like quick with how fast you move from exercise to exercise in each circuit in this workout—a great push for your mind and body.

CIRCUIT 1

EXERCISE	DURATION	PAGE
One-armed dumbbell row	6 reps	138
Squat jumps	6 reps	98
Single-armed kettlebell carry	8 reps	50
Rest	90 secs	

CIRCUIT 2

EXERCISE	DURATION	PAGE
Handstand pushups	8 reps	74
Overhead slams	6 reps	78
Jumping knees	4 reps per side	108
Rest	90 secs	

CIRCUIT 3

EXERCISE	DURATION	PAGE
Elbow taps	12 reps	38
Glute march	12 reps	72
Kettlebell punches	20 secs	42
Rest	90 secs	

180   Power Program

Exercises are listed with page numbers for easy reference

PROGRAMS

Three programs—focused on developing strength, power, or stability—combine workouts for daily, weekly, and monthly progressions to push you toward developing a fighter's physique.

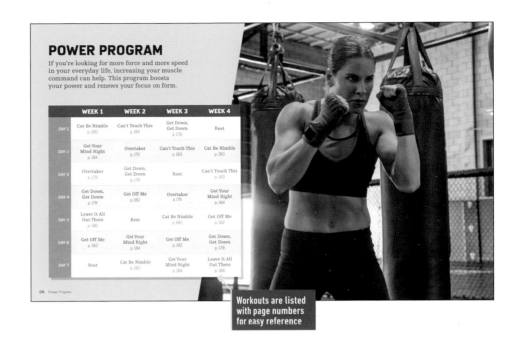

POWER PROGRAM

If you're looking for more force and more speed in your everyday life, increasing your muscle command can help. This program boosts your power and renews your focus on form.

	WEEK 1	WEEK 2	WEEK 3	WEEK 4
DAY 1	Cat Be Nimble p. 180	Can't Touch This p. 183	Get Down, Get Down p. 178	Rest
DAY 2	Get Your Mind Right p. 184	Overtaker p. 179	Can't Touch This p. 183	Cat Be Nimble p. 180
DAY 3	Overtaker p. 179	Get Down, Get Down p. 178	Rest	Can't Touch This p. 183
DAY 4	Get Down, Get Down p. 178	Get Off Me p. 182	Overtaker p. 179	Get Your Mind Right p. 184
DAY 5	Leave It All Out There p. 186	Rest	Cat Be Nimble p. 180	Get Off Me p. 182
DAY 6	Get Off Me p. 182	Get Your Mind Right p. 184	Get Off Me p. 182	Get Down, Get Down p. 178
DAY 7	Rest	Cat Be Nimble p. 180	Get Your Mind Right p. 184	Leave It All Out There p. 186

176 Power Program

Workouts are listed with page numbers for easy reference

Common MMA disciplines

Boxing If you think boxing is all about punching, then you're missing out on its other aspects, including developing strong footwork and core muscles.

Brazilian jiu-jitsu This is a somewhat down-and-dirty style that can help you develop agility from many different positions—on the ground or standing up—because you'll use different muscles on the ground from when you're standing.

Judo Focused mostly on throwing and grappling, this form has developed into a combat style of fighting.

Many exercises in this book include judo techniques.

Karate This style is heavy on striking moves, but it's also one of the core elements of kickboxing. Several exercises in this book are good conditioning for the karate discipline.

Kickboxing With a foundation of kicking and punching (thus the name), this style can offer a complete workout, which is why some exercises in this book involve kicks and strikes.

Muay Thai This style offers a full-body workout because it's

all about legs, knees, elbows, and fists, which is why this discipline compares well with kickboxing, which uses most of the same kinds of muscle areas.

Taekwondo This style incorporates elements of karate and kung-fu, especially various kicking elements. Some exercises in this book match well with this style.

Wrestling Like with boxing, this style helps train your body for better movement and better stamina. You'll spend some time on the ground in this book, and this style is an influence.

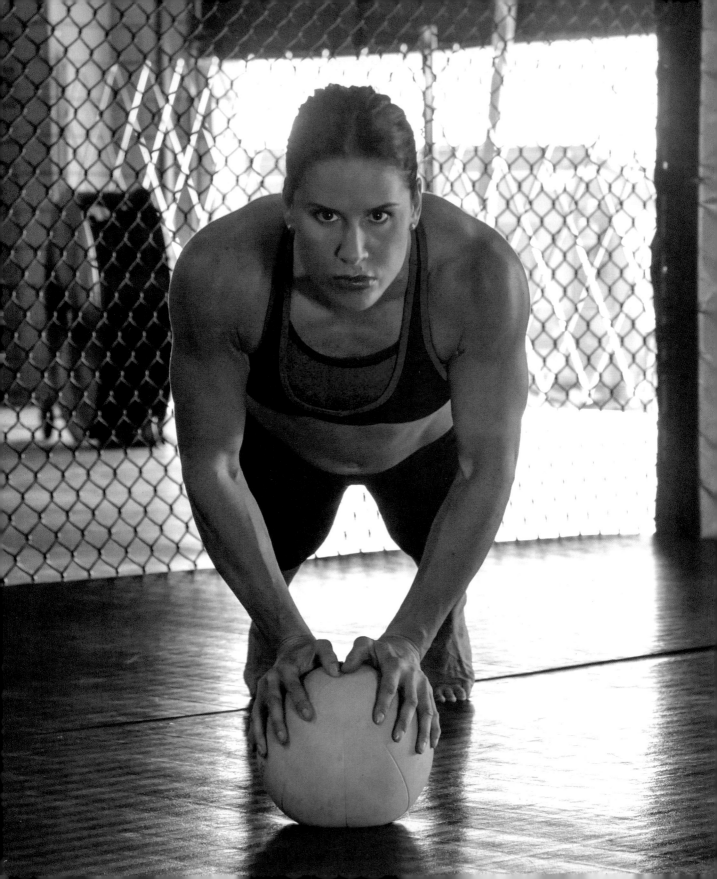

UPPER-BODY EXERCISES

MEDICINE BALL PUNCHES

Launching a medicine ball against a wall not only feels amazing on the inside, but it makes for a speedy and dynamic contribution to your strikes and reaction times. The twist also engages all parts of your power muscles.

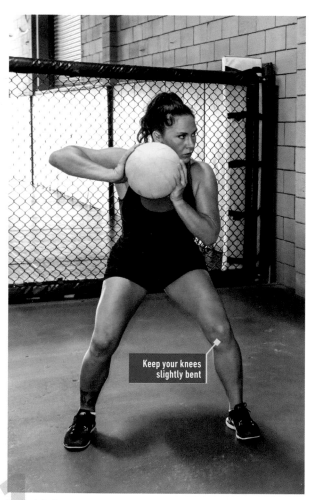

Keep your knees slightly bent

Stand 3 feet away from a wall, with your left side facing the wall, put your legs wider than hip-width apart, and hold a medicine ball in your hands at your chest.

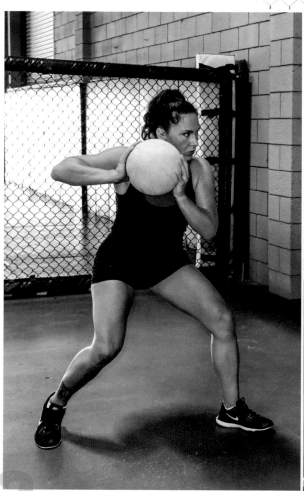

Bend your right knee as you slightly step forward, opening your stance and turning your right hip toward the wall.

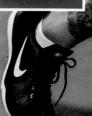

3 Extend your right arm in front of you, initiating the throw with your lower body, and throw the ball toward the wall, finishing with the extension of your upper body. Reach out with both hands to catch the rebound, then return to your starting position. Repeat steps 2 and 3 for the duration listed in a workout, then switch sides.

MAKE IT **HARDER**

In step 1, start farther away from the wall. In step 2, add a twist from the hips before catching the ball—switching the way you twist with each throw.

TARGETS /// upper back, arms, abs, lower back, obliques, quads, glutes, and hamstrings
EQUIPMENT /// none

TEMPO PUSHUPS

These pushups are about being slow and with the intention of controlling each engaged muscle. Being deliberate about poise and posture creates a strengthening burn that impacts your whole body.

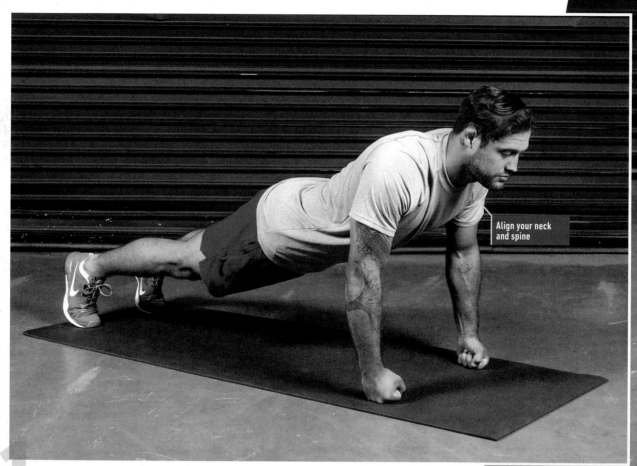

Align your neck and spine

Put your fists on the ground, with your legs hip-width apart, and balance your body on the tips of your toes.

MAKE IT HARDER

In step 2, hold the up position and the down position for 3 seconds each for an even stronger resistance.

Keep your shoulders over your wrists

2 Bend your elbows to slowly lower yourself to the ground, then reverse your movements to return to your starting position. Repeat this step for the duration listed in a workout.

TARGETS /// shoulders, chest, triceps, and abs
EQUIPMENT /// dumbbells

FLOOR PRESS

Lifting while on the ground provides a practical position to MMA, where strength and push are vital. Forming and maintaining these explosive motions create tight and consistent power in your core and upper body.

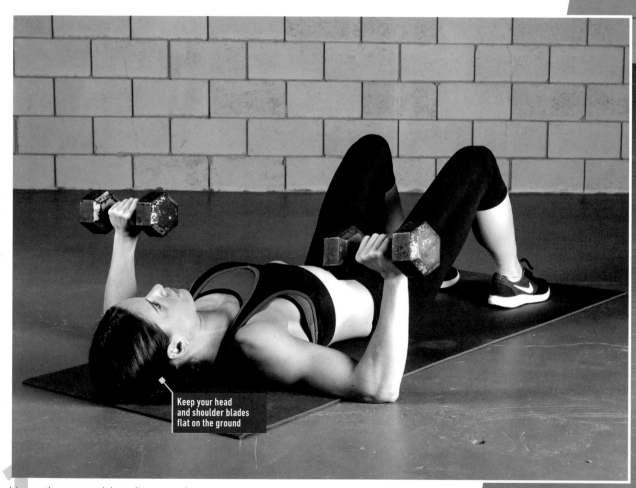

Keep your head and shoulder blades flat on the ground

Lie on the ground, bending your knees and keeping your feet flat on the ground. Hold dumbbells in each hand at your chest, forming 90° angles with your arms and keeping your upper arms flat on the ground.

Push through your tailbone to help you lift the dumbbells

MAKE IT HARDER

In step 2, hold the dumbbells in your extended arms for 5 seconds, then take 5 seconds to return to your starting position.

Push the dumbbells up with explosive force, keeping a slight bend in your elbows. Reverse your movements and slowly return to your starting position. Repeat this step for the duration listed in a workout.

MEDICINE BALL CHEST PRESS

Training this chest press with a medicine ball means engaging your core and developing your explosive strength, coordination, and dexterity. Control the ball— and control your results.

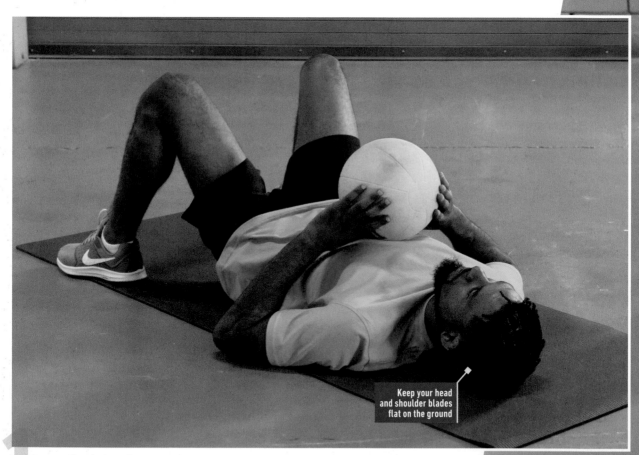

Keep your head and shoulder blades flat on the ground

Lie on your back, bending your knees and keeping your feet flat on the ground. Hold a medicine ball in both hands at your chest, keeping the backs of your arms flat on the ground.

Toss the ball only a few inches beyond your reach

Keep your arms extended until you catch the ball

Explode and extend your arms straight up as you release the ball directly above your chest. Catch the ball as it comes back down, then repeat this step for the duration listed in a workout.

TARGETS /// back, shoulders, abs, and legs
EQUIPMENT /// none

ELBOW TAPS

This exercise forces you to stabilize and control your entire posture, creating a tightening effect as you hold the position and work all target areas simultaneously. This is also a test of your flexibility and dexterity.

1 Put your hands flat on the ground, pointing your fingers forward, and balance your body on the balls of your feet.

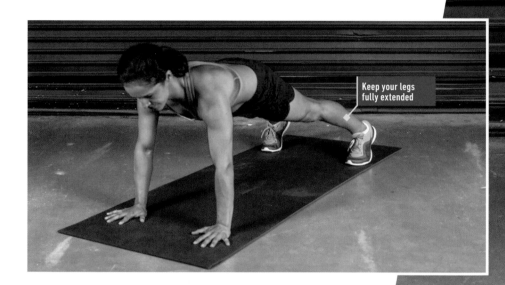

Keep your legs fully extended

2 Bend your right elbow to reach your right arm across your body to touch your left elbow with your right hand, then reverse your movements to return to your starting position.

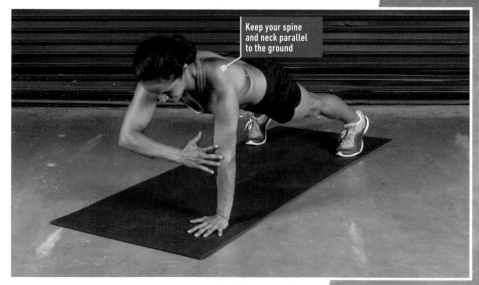

Keep your spine and neck parallel to the ground

Keep your weight from shifting from side to side

MAKE IT HARDER

In steps 2 and 3, touch your right knee to your left elbow and touch your left knee to your right elbow.

Bend your left elbow to reach your left arm across your body to touch your inner right elbow with your left hand, then reverse your movements to return to your starting position. Repeat steps 2 and 3 for the duration listed in a workout.

TARGETS /// shoulders, back, biceps, and triceps
EQUIPMENT /// none

ARM CIRCLES

This motion creates an isometric burn throughout your trapezoids, shoulders, and lats. Strengthening these areas decreases potential fatigue, especially during those later stages of a workout circuit.

1 Stand with your feet shoulder-width apart and extend your arms at your sides until they're perpendicular to your body. Begin to draw circles with your arms, catching at the bottom and the top of the rotation.

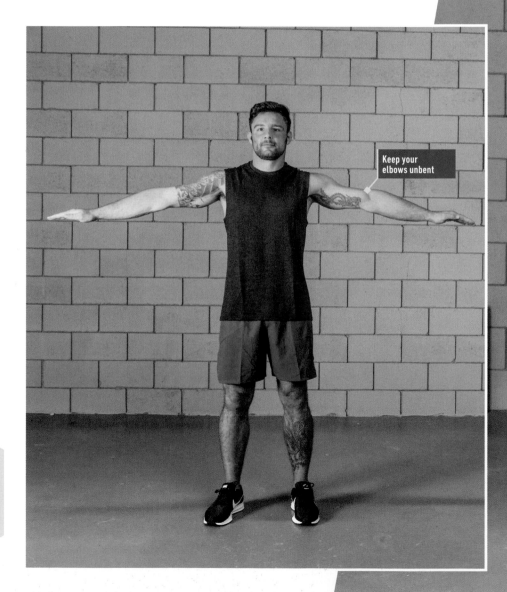

Keep your elbows unbent

TIP
Creating slower circles can increase the results you feel.

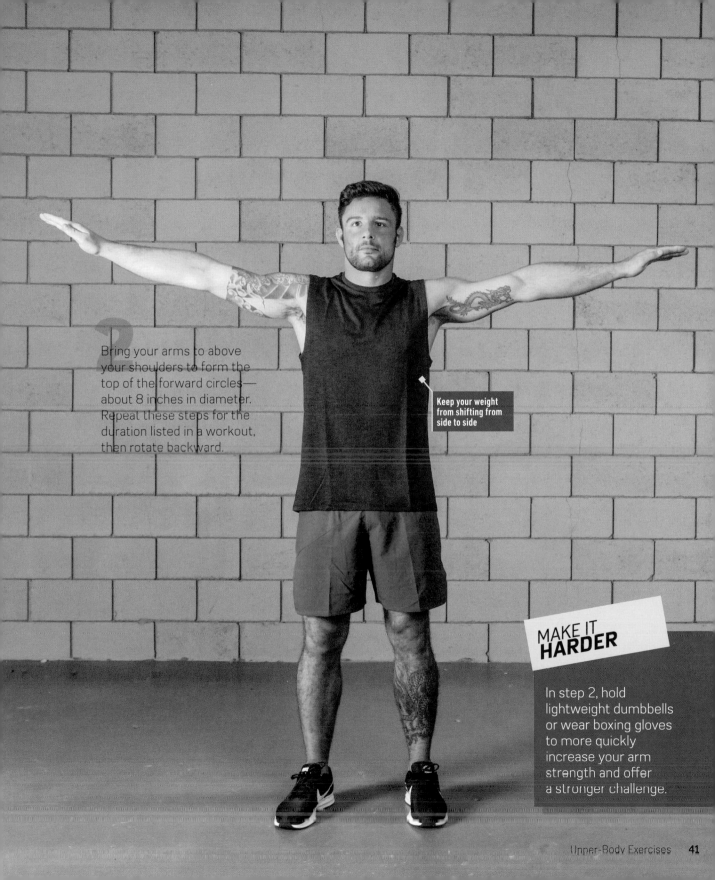

2 Bring your arms to above your shoulders to form the top of the forward circles—about 8 inches in diameter. Repeat these steps for the duration listed in a workout, then rotate backward.

Keep your weight from shifting from side to side

MAKE IT HARDER

In step 2, hold lightweight dumbbells or wear boxing gloves to more quickly increase your arm strength and offer a stronger challenge.

KETTLEBELL PUNCHES

If you're looking for an exercise to tone your upper body, this explosive exercise works wonders. You'll also develop balanced symmetry through rotational movement, helping with shoulder stability and hand-eye coordination.

1

Stand with your feet wider than hip-width apart, hold a kettlebell in your right hand, and extend your arm out in front of you. As you exchange arms, bring your knuckles back to your face.

Keep your knees slightly bent

TIP
Start with a lightweight kettlebell until this becomes too easy.

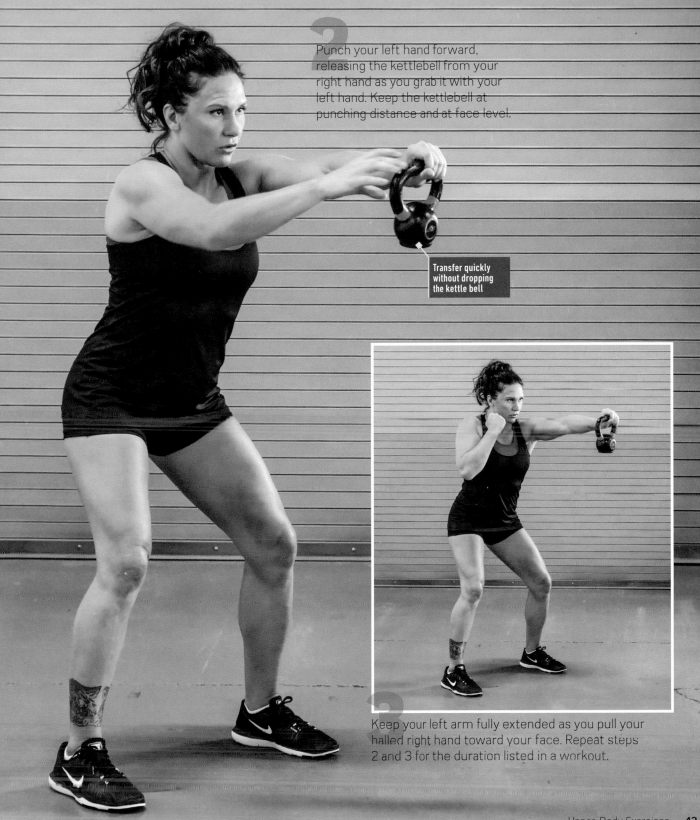

2 Punch your left hand forward, releasing the kettlebell from your right hand as you grab it with your left hand. Keep the kettlebell at punching distance and at face level.

Transfer quickly without dropping the kettle bell

3 Keep your left arm fully extended as you pull your halled right hand toward your face. Repeat steps 2 and 3 for the duration listed in a workout.

ONE-ARMED PRESS

Performing this exercise benefits you in ways typical two-armed exercises can't: increasing core stability, putting muscles under tension for longer individual time periods, and developing better isometric control.

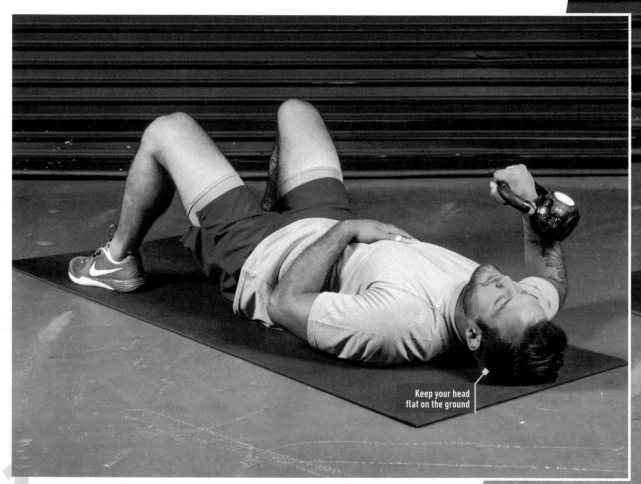

Keep your head flat on the ground

Lie on your back, bending your knees and keeping your feet flat on the ground. Hold a kettlebell in your right hand above your right shoulder, and rest your left hand on your stomach.

In step 2, after you've fully extended your arm, hold the kettlebell in place for 5 seconds for each rep.

Press your tailbone into the ground as you lift the kettlebell

Push the kettlebell straight up until your elbow is extended directly above your shoulder, keeping the kettlebell at shoulder level, then reverse your movements to return to your starting position. Repeat this step for the duration listed in a workout, then switch sides.

TARGETS /// arms, shoulders, abs, and glutes
EQUIPMENT /// barbell plate

PLATE DROPS

This drop-and-catch motion forces your fast twitch and muscle memory to ignite, creating a burn throughout your body—from head to toe.

1 Stand with your feet wider than hip-width apart and hold a barbell plate in both hands, extending your arms out in front of you at face level.

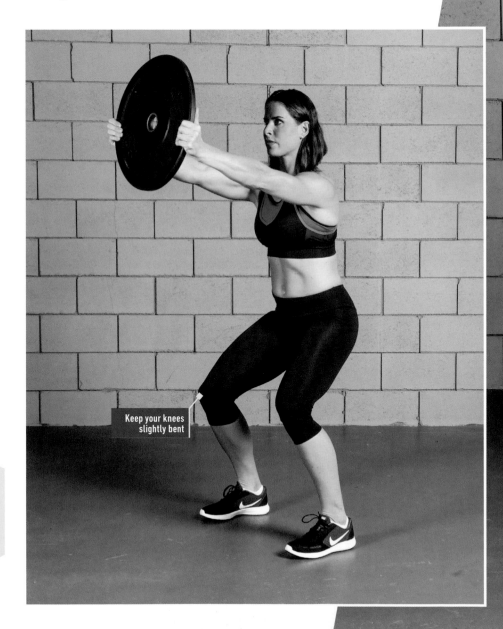

Keep your knees slightly bent

TIP
Use a lighter weight to help you focus on form—and see quick results.

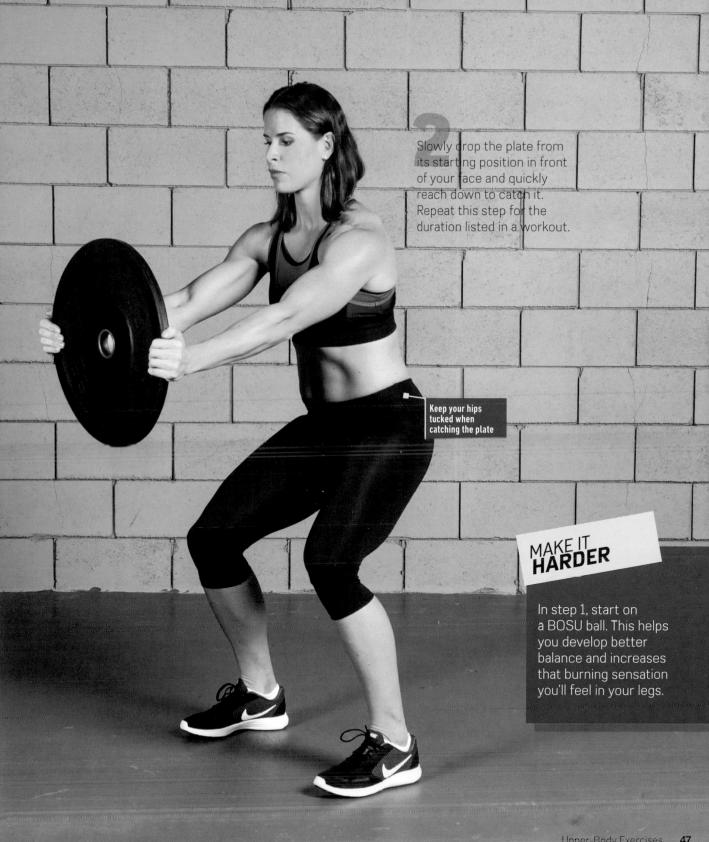

2 Slowly drop the plate from its starting position in front of your face and quickly reach down to catch it. Repeat this step for the duration listed in a workout.

Keep your hips tucked when catching the plate

MAKE IT **HARDER**

In step 1, start on a BOSU ball. This helps you develop better balance and increases that burning sensation you'll feel in your legs.

MEDICINE BALL SITUPS

This situps version forces you to perform them in dynamic and engaging ways that tests your physical limits—but gives you amazing rewards and a new look at what it takes to develop core strength.

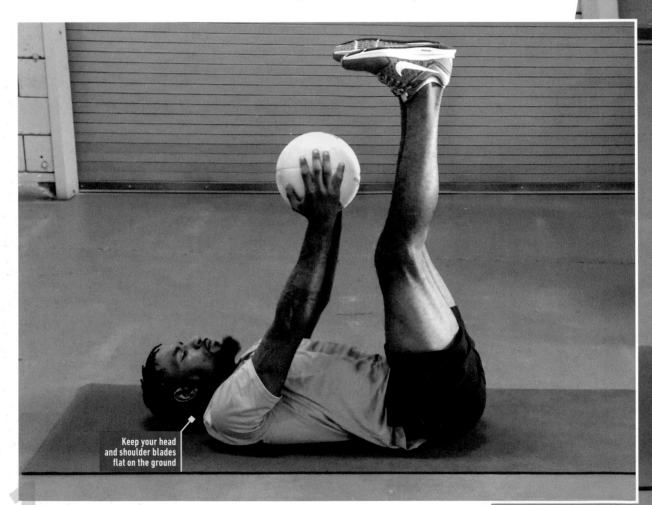

Keep your head and shoulder blades flat on the ground

Lie on your back, extending your legs and arms straight up, and hold a medicine ball in your hands directly above your chest, keeping your chin tucked.

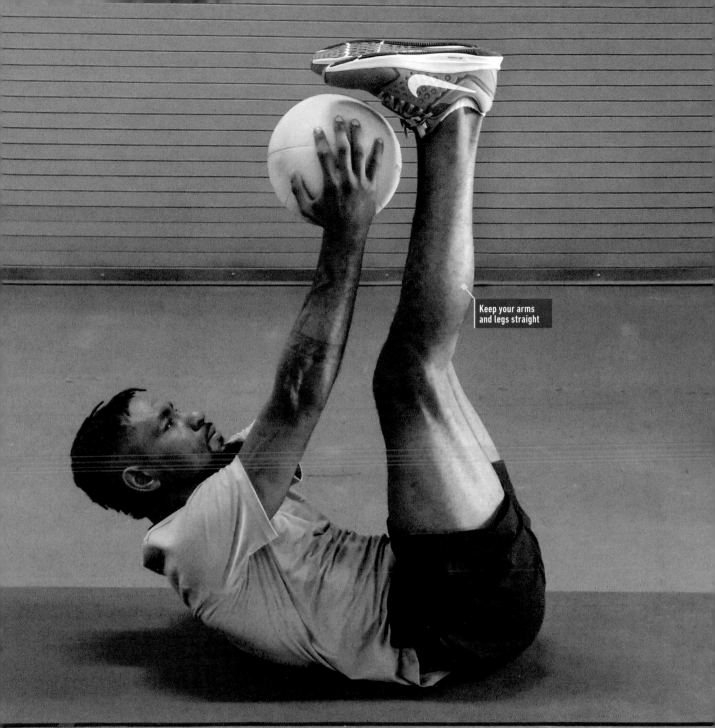

Keep your arms and legs straight

Lift your upper back off the ground and reach the ball toward your toes, flexing your feet. Reverse your movements to return to your starting position, then repeat this step for the duration listed in a workout.

ONE-ARMED KETTLEBELL CARRY

This exercise encourages you to develop stability and balance by focusing on one arm at a time and switching arms while still in motion. You'll also work on your posture and agility.

1 Stand with your feet hip-width apart, holding a kettlebell in your right hand, then step your left foot forward.

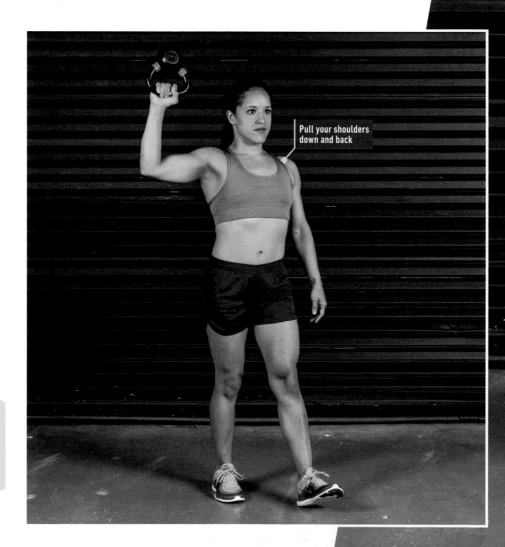

Pull your shoulders down and back

TIP
Engage your abs during the carry to better develop your core.

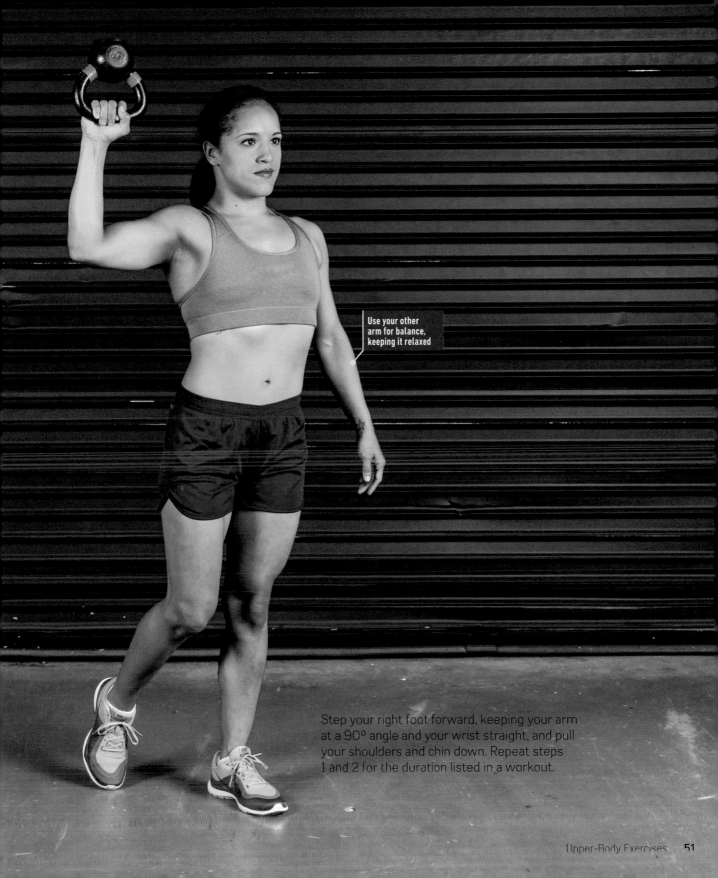

Use your other arm for balance, keeping it relaxed

Step your right foot forward, keeping your arm at a 90º angle and your wrist straight, and pull your shoulders and chin down. Repeat steps 1 and 2 for the duration listed in a workout.

TARGETS /// arms, shoulders, abs, hamstrings, and calves
EQUIPMENT /// kettlebell

ONE-LEGGED WEIGHT DROPS

Keeping your balance is essential to performing everyday activities. This exercise can develop those muscles responsible for helping you maintain your balance, strengthening your glutes, hamstrings, and shoulders.

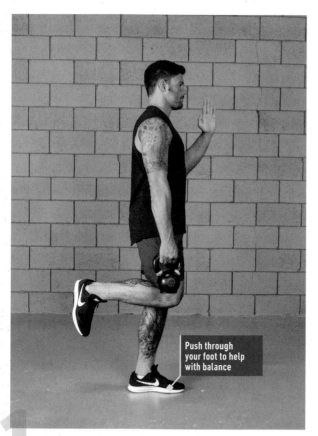

Push through your foot to help with balance

1 Stand with your feet slightly apart, holding a kettlebell in your right hand at your knee and raising your left hand to just above your shoulder. Bend your right knee and extend your right leg behind you to form a 90° angle.

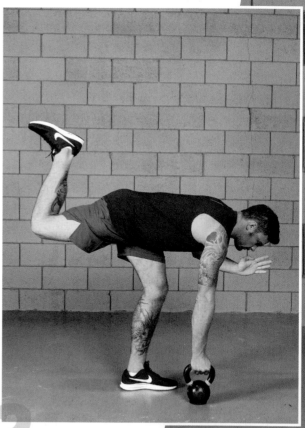

2 Bend at your hips to fully extend your right arm and lower the kettlebell to the ground.

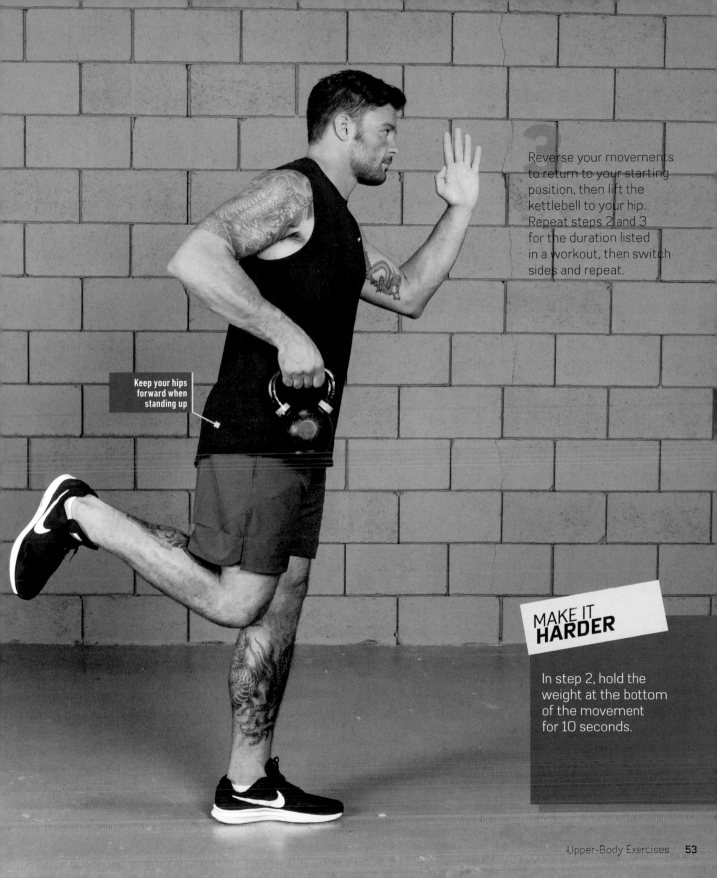

3 Reverse your movements to return to your starting position, then lift the kettlebell to your hip. Repeat steps 2 and 3 for the duration listed in a workout, then switch sides and repeat.

Keep your hips forward when standing up

MAKE IT **HARDER**

In step 2, hold the weight at the bottom of the movement for 10 seconds.

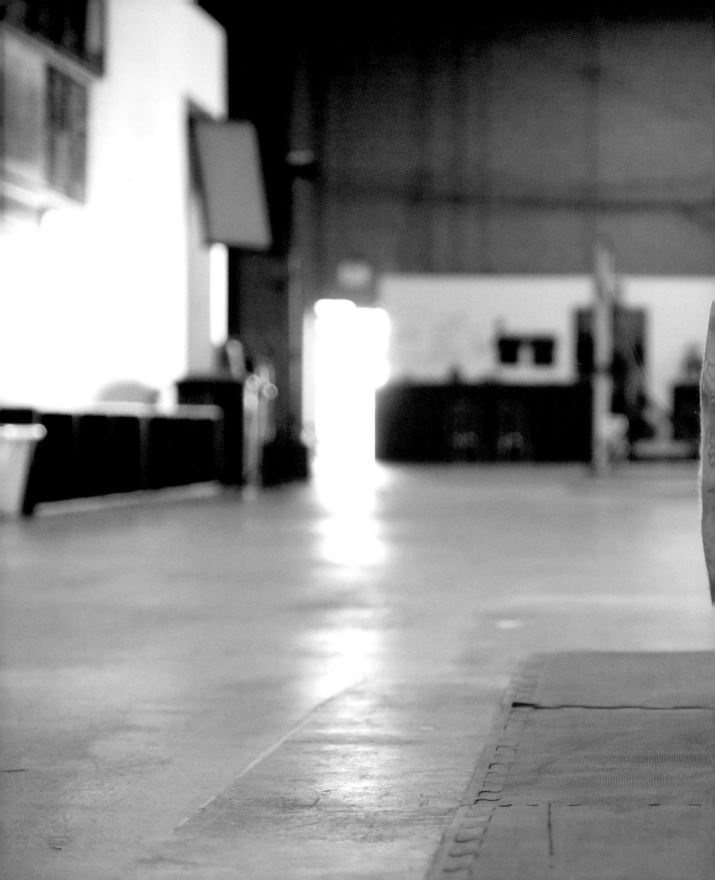

CORE EXERCISES

TARGETS /// shoulders, abs, and glutes
EQUIPMENT /// none

KNEE-TO-ELBOW TOUCHES

Developing and strengthening the stabilizing muscles in your shoulders, abdomen, and hip flexors during this exercise can give you the foundation for enhancing the rest of your body's muscles.

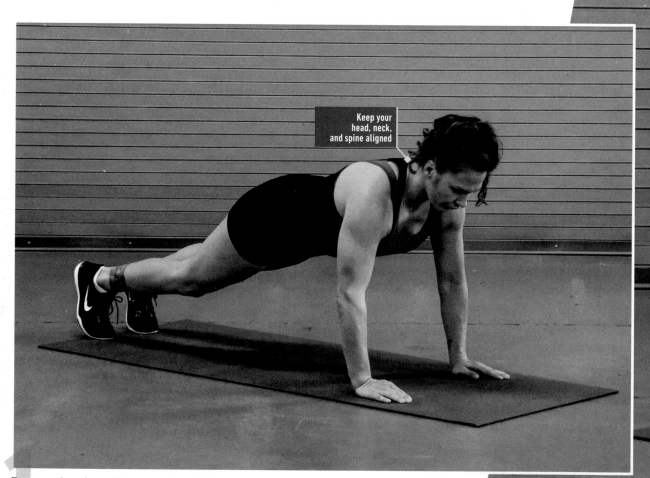

Keep your head, neck, and spine aligned

1 Put your hands on the ground, pointing your fingers forward, and balance your legs on the balls of your toes. Keep your spine and neck parallel to the ground and keep your chin tucked.

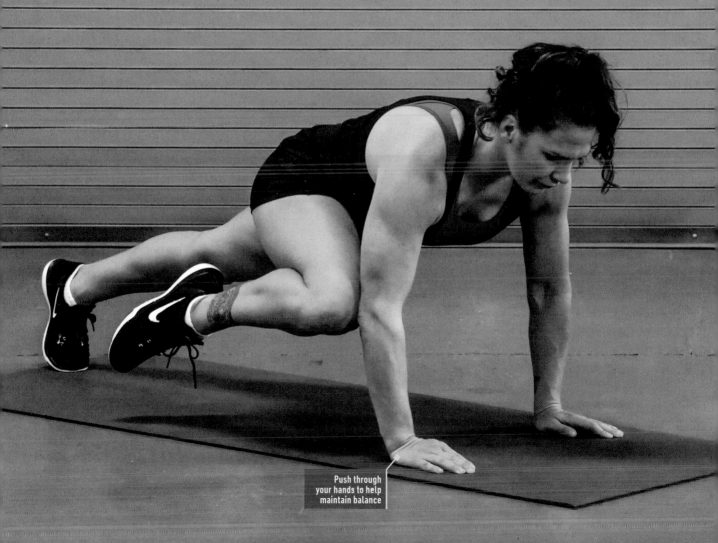

TIP
Keep your weight centered and your hips slightly tucked for optimal exertion.

2
Lift your right leg off the ground and bend your right knee as you bring your right knee to touch your right elbow, then reverse your movements to return to your starting position. Repeat this step for the duration listed in a workout, then switch legs.

Push through your hands to help maintain balance

PLANK DROP TO ELBOWS

Work your balance, strength, and stability in motion, maintaining your position while manipulating your base. Feel that constant tug on your core, and push against gravity for an even more powerful experience.

1 Put your hands flat on the ground, pointing your fingers forward, and balance your weight on the tips of your toes, forming the classic pushup position.

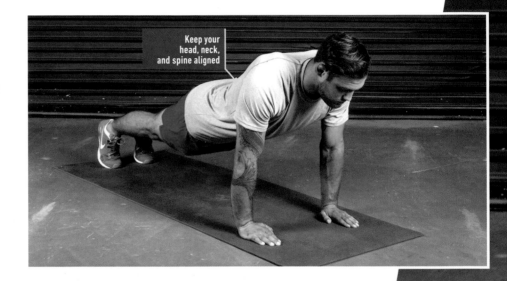

Keep your head, neck, and spine aligned

2 Bend your right elbow to place your right forearm on the ground, facing your right hand palm up, keeping your left hand flat on the ground, and slightly bending your left elbow.

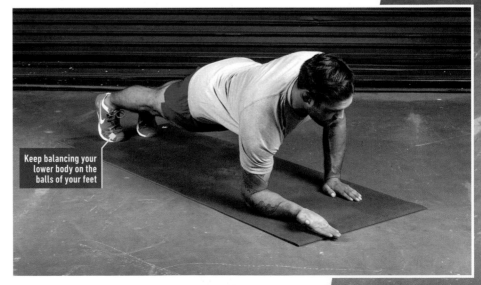

Keep balancing your lower body on the balls of your feet

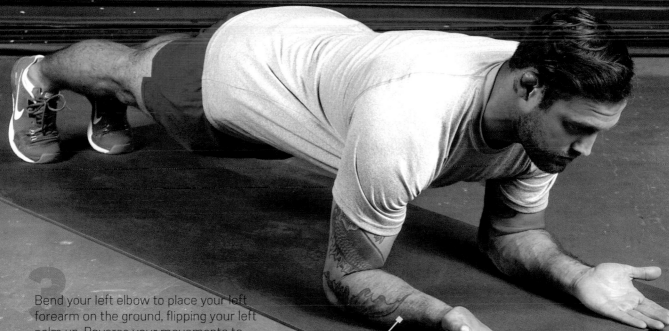

TIP
Keep your hips
tucked and your
palms up for
optimal burn.

3

Bend your left elbow to place your left
forearm on the ground, flipping your left
palm up. Reverse your movements to
return to your starting pushup position,
then repeat steps 2 and 3 for the
duration listed in a workout.

**Push through your
forearms to help
with balance**

TARGETS /// chest, biceps, triceps, abs, and obliques
EQUIPMENT /// T-shirt

T-SHIRT CURLS

Isometric exercises like this one are static, meaning joint angle and muscle length don't change during contractions. But your continuous motions can give you a burn you weren't expecting!

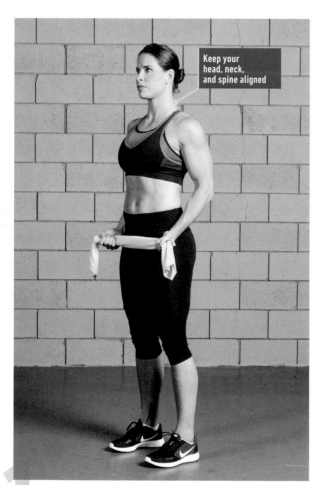

Keep your head, neck, and spine aligned

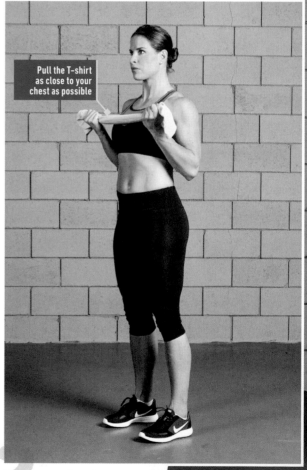

Pull the T-shirt as close to your chest as possible

1 Stand with your feet hip-width apart and hold a rolled-up T-shirt in your hands in front of your hips, placing your hands 1 foot apart on the T-shirt.

2 Bend your elbows as you lift the T-shirt toward your chest, keeping the T-shirt taut between your hands and keeping your elbows tight to your ribs.

3 Reach your arms above your head, fully extending your arms, then reverse your movements to return to your starting position. Repeat steps 2 and 3 for the duration listed in a workout.

Engage your core when you reach your arms over your head

MAKE IT **HARDER**

In step 1, start on your knees and use a heavier weight. Or in step 2, perform a lunge or a step-up during the hold period.

TARGETS /// abs, back, and hips
EQUIPMENT /// none

BIRD DOG

Balance, flexion, and contraction are important in all aspects of exercising and toning the core. Isolating one side at a time adds a great challenge while you're alternating crunching and straightening your body.

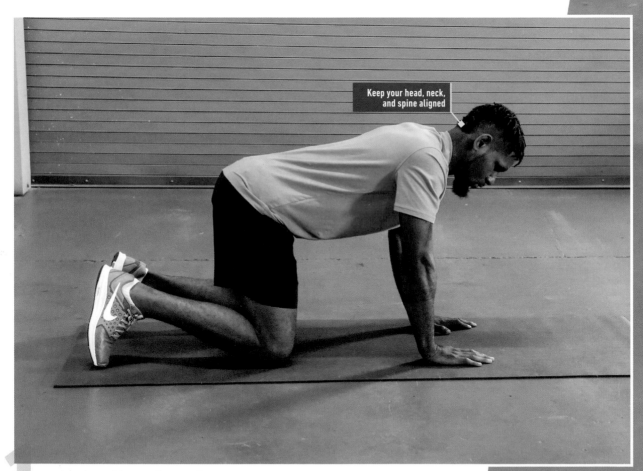

Keep your head, neck, and spine aligned

1 Put your hands and knees flat on the ground, pointing your fingers forward and forming 90° angles with your legs. Keep your spine and neck parallel to the ground and keep your chin tucked.

Lift your right leg and your left arm off the ground, then bend your left elbow as you bring your right knee toward your left elbow until they touch underneath your abdomen.

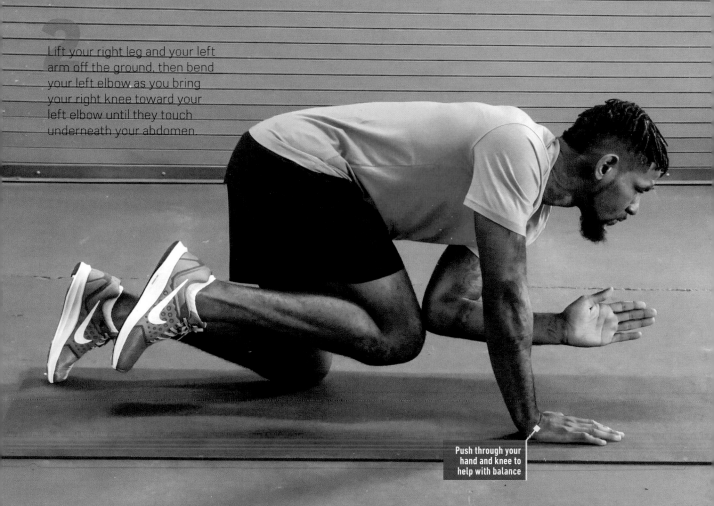

Push through your hand and knee to help with balance

Extend your right leg behind you, flexing your foot to engage your leg muscles, and extend your left arm in front of you until they're parallel with the ground. Reverse your movements to return to your starting position. Repeat steps 2 and 3 for the duration listed in a workout, then switch sides.

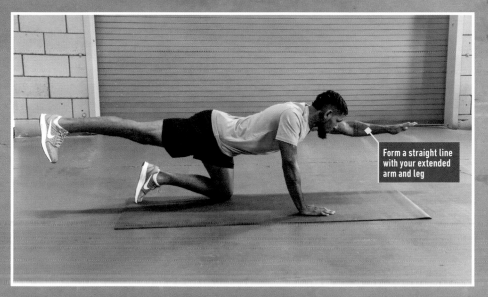

Form a straight line with your extended arm and leg

TARGETS **///** groin, abs, calves, glutes, hamstrings, hip flexors, obliques, thighs, and quads
EQUIPMENT **///** none

CARIOCA (SIDE-TO-SIDE STEPS)

This samba variation includes aspects of calisthenics, cardio, and stretching, invigorating blood flow to the joints and letting you develop and utilize different muscle groups and footwork via lateral dance-like motions.

1

Stand with your feet hip-width apart and relax your arms at your sides.

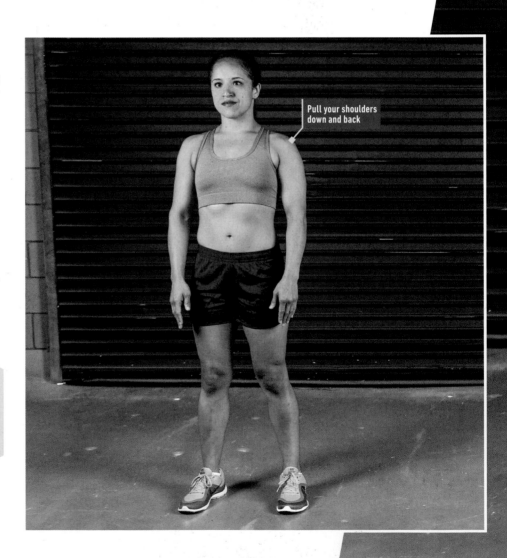

Pull your shoulders down and back

TIP
Exaggerate lifting the front knee for optimal flexion and coordination.

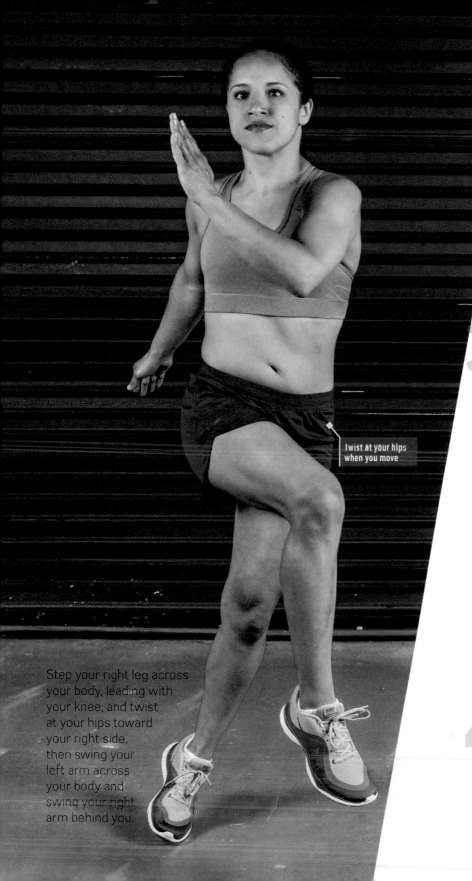

Twist at your hips when you move

Step your right leg across your body, leading with your knee, and twist at your hips toward your right side, then swing your left arm across your body and swing your right arm behind you.

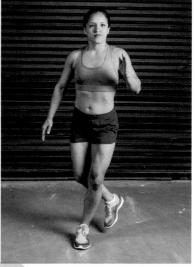

Plant your right foot on the ground, then step your left leg behind you. Cross your right foot over and in front of your left foot, then cross your left foot over and in front of your right foot.

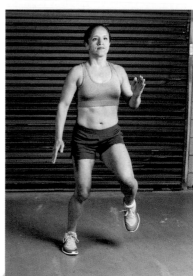

Cross your right foot over and in front of your left foot, then cross your left foot over and in front of your right foot. Repeat steps 2 to 4 for the duration listed in a workout.

TARGETS /// hamstrings, abs, obliques, and hip flexors
EQUIPMENT /// medicine ball

MEDICINE BALL TWIST

Keeping your legs elevated while rotating your upper body challenges your mind and midsection. Focus on consistent rhythm and balance, and watch yourself fly through these twists.

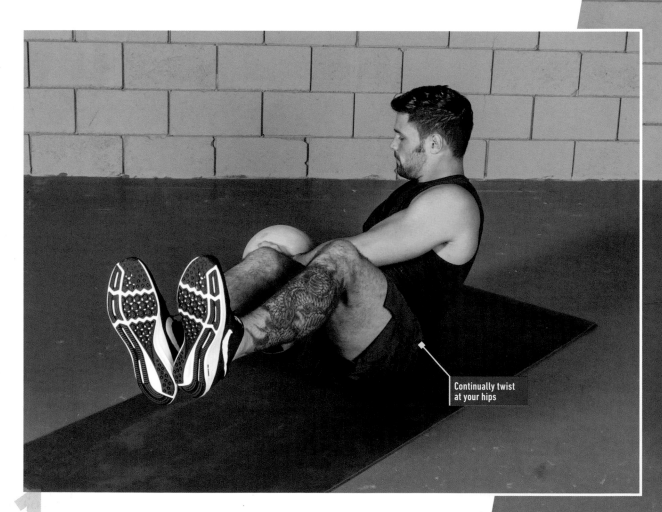

Continually twist at your hips

1 Sit on the ground in a comfortable position, raising your legs off the ground and holding a medicine ball at your midsection. Twist at your hips to touch the ground by your right hip with the ball.

2 Twist at your hips to swing the ball
across your body toward your left
hip, touching the ball to the ground.
Repeat steps 2 and 3 for the duration
listed in a workout.

TARGETS **///** quads, calves, and hamstrings
EQUIPMENT **///** plyometric box

BOX JUMPS

This exercise might have you thinking "legs," when
in fact it's core engagement that gets you on the box.
Once you've stuck the landing, then your legs take over
to help you complete the move as you stand tall at the top.

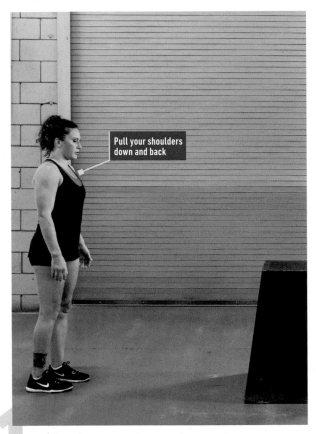

Pull your shoulders down and back

1 Stand a few feet away from a plyometric box, keeping your feet hip-width apart and relaxing your arms at your sides.

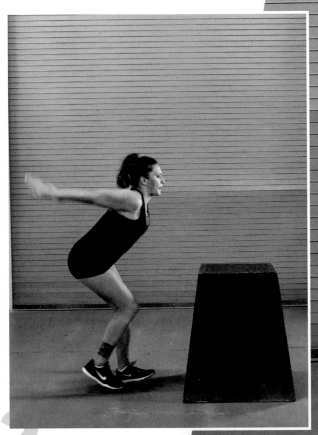

2 Take two quick steps toward the box, bringing your feet together 1 foot in front of the box to initiate takeoff, then swing your arms behind you and bend your knees as you prepare to jump.

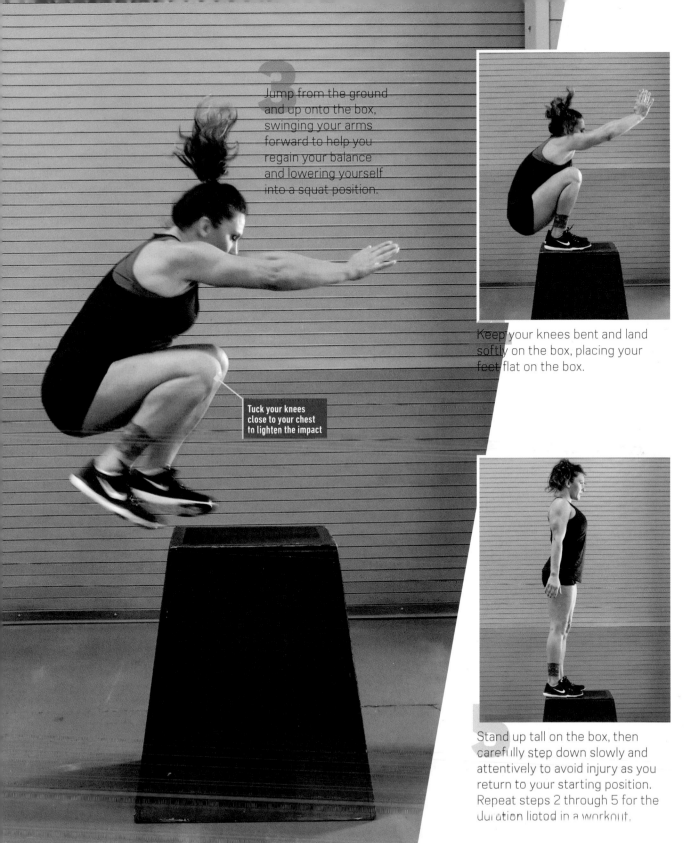

3 Jump from the ground and up onto the box, swinging your arms forward to help you regain your balance and lowering yourself into a squat position.

Tuck your knees close to your chest to lighten the impact

Keep your knees bent and land softly on the box, placing your feet flat on the box.

Stand up tall on the box, then carefully step down slowly and attentively to avoid injury as you return to your starting position. Repeat steps 2 through 5 for the duration listed in a workout.

KETTLEBELL PULLS

Bodyweight exercises can help you strengthen and tone your upper body, and adding weights to a bodyweight exercise can challenge you differently and more efficiently.

1

Place your hands flat on the ground, centered under your shoulders, and balance your weight on the balls of your feet. Place a kettlebell on the ground behind your left hand and at rib level.

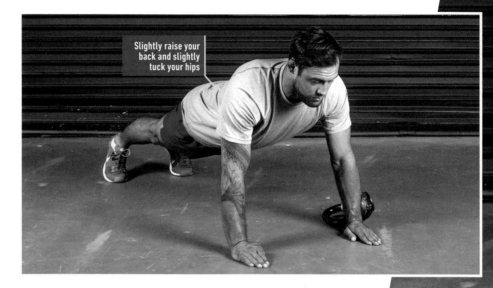

Slightly raise your back and slightly tuck your hips

2

Reach your right arm across your body to grab the kettlebell with your right hand, beginning to drag it from behind your left hand.

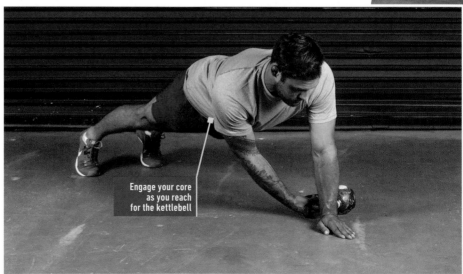

Engage your core as you reach for the kettlebell

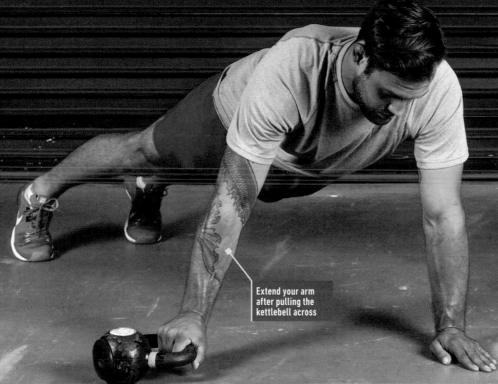

TIP
Keep your weight from shifting, engaging your core for balance.

Extend your arm after pulling the kettlebell across

Pull the kettlebell across the floor until your right hand reaches its starting position, then swing it to face the handle in to prepare for the other hand.

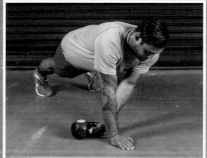

Reach your left arm across your body to grab the kettlebell with your left hand, pulling it across the floor until your left hand reaches its starting position. Repeat steps 2 and 3 for the duration listed in a workout.

TARGETS /// triceps, glutes, hamstrings, and core
EQUIPMENT /// none

GLUTE MARCH

This bridge variation can improve hamstring and quad mobility and strengthen your lower back and glutes. This exercise can also tighten your core muscles—ideal for looking like a fighter!

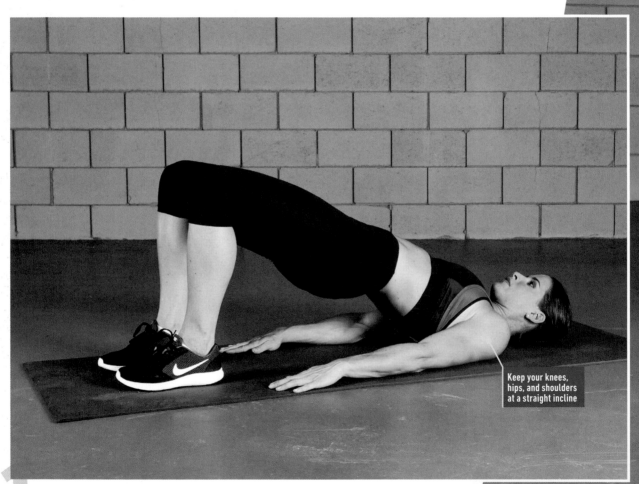

Keep your knees, hips, and shoulders at a straight incline

1 Lie on your back, bending your knees, keeping your feet flat on the ground, and relaxing your arms at your sides. Press your heels into the ground to lift your lower back off the ground.

2 Lift your left leg off the ground, fully extending it and keeping it on the same plane as the grounded leg, then reverse your movements to return to your starting position—but keep your lower back lifted off the ground. Repeat this step for the duration listed in a workout, then switch legs.

Keep your hips and back elevated

MAKE IT HARDER

In step 1, add weights around your ankles to enhance the impact on your legs.

HANDSTAND PUSHUPS

This exercise strengthens your triceps for arm extensions, your shoulders for overhead actions, and your pectorals for forward thrusts—all of which increase your power and agility when performing boxing or grappling moves.

1 Place a foam block close to a wall, then face that wall. Place your hands evenly on both sides of the block, then kick your legs up and back so you're facing away from the wall.

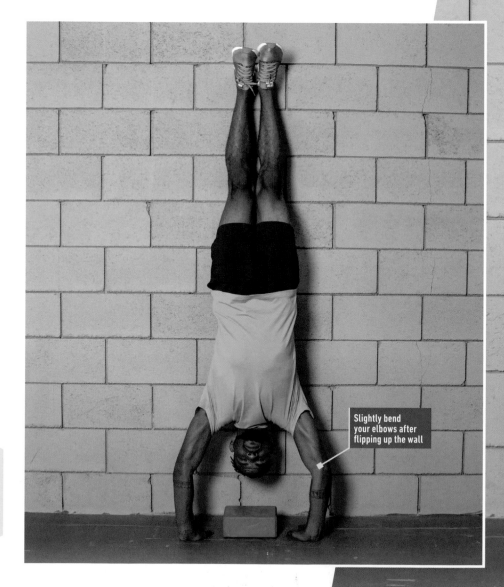

Slightly bend your elbows after flipping up the wall

TIP
Stay focused on your form to push yourself through the fatigue.

2 Bend your elbows to slowly lower yourself down, stopping when your head touches the block. Reverse your movements to return to your starting position, then repeat this step for the duration listed in a workout.

Engage your core to help you maintain balance

MAKE IT HARDER

In step 1, use a smaller block for your head. In step 2, perform the reps faster.

MEDICINE BALL HIP THROWS

Small deliberate motions can benefit you and your physicality in your everyday training. How close you stand to the wall in this exercise can increase your physicality, mental flexibility, and reaction times.

1

Stand with your left side slightly facing a wall, putting your right foot a few feet in front of your left foot and slightly squatting, and hold a medicine ball at your right hip.

TIP
Squatting makes the twist shorter and the throw more effective.

Push through the balls of your feet and recoil at the hips

2 Slightly twist at your hips until more of your upper body faces the wall, then quickly release the ball against the wall, catching the rebound and recoiling back to your starting position. Repeat this step for the duration listed in a workout.

Keep your palms open for more catching control

MAKE IT HARDER

In step 2, step and twist away from the wall and change the target vertically with each rep.

TARGETS /// back, shoulders, core, glutes, and legs
EQUIPMENT /// medicine ball

OVERHEAD SLAMS

In fighting, you commonly see someone get snapped from standing on their feet straight to being face down on the ground. This exercise simulates a motion that creates a force so strong that your core strength is unstoppable.

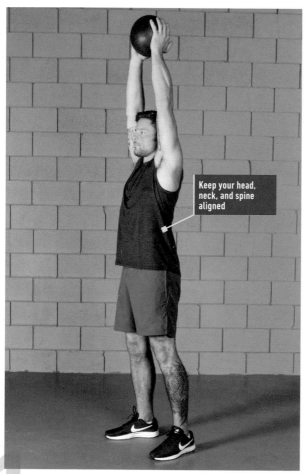

Keep your head, neck, and spine aligned

1 Stand with your feet hip-width apart and hold a medicine ball in both hands directly over your head.

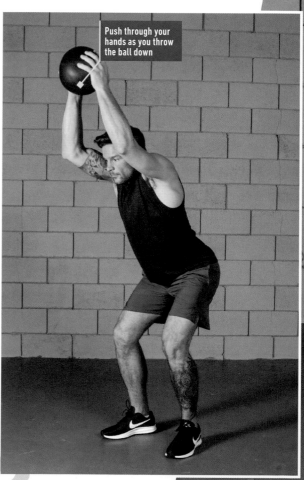

Push through your hands as you throw the ball down

2 Use gravity as you bend at the hips and the ball drops, gaining momentum, then push the ball with 100% force into the ground from the top of the ball.

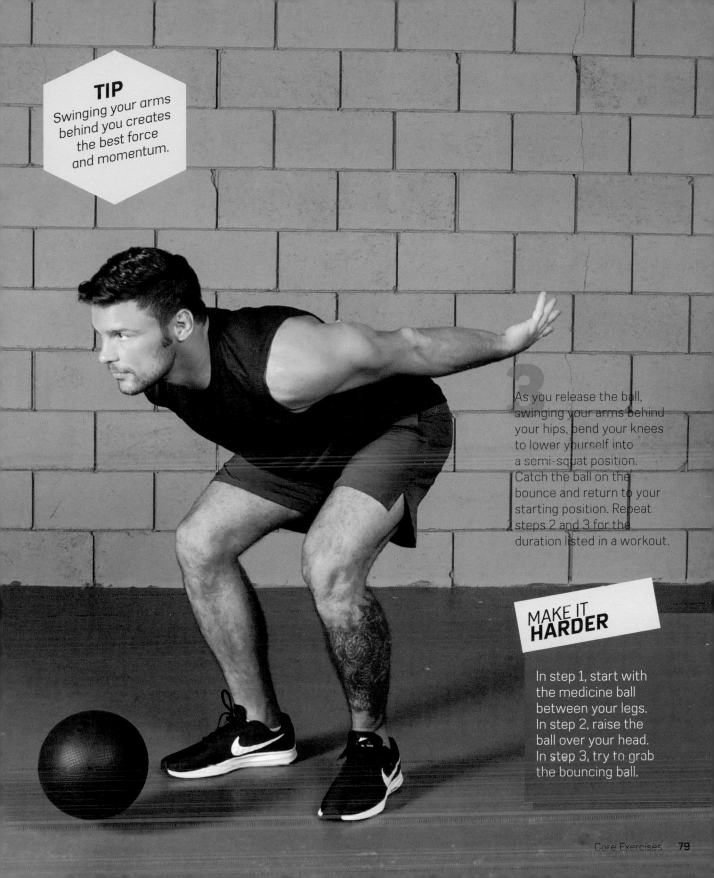

TIP
Swinging your arms behind you creates the best force and momentum.

As you release the ball, swinging your arms behind your hips, bend your knees to lower yourself into a semi-squat position. Catch the ball on the bounce and return to your starting position. Repeat steps 2 and 3 for the duration listed in a workout.

MAKE IT HARDER

In step 1, start with the medicine ball between your legs. In step 2, raise the ball over your head. In step 3, try to grab the bouncing ball.

TARGETS /// glutes, calves, and quads
EQUIPMENT /// medicine ball

MEDICINE BALL WALL SIT

Pressing your body into a wall and pressing your hands into a ball create resistance in your legs and arms. The burn and quiver you feel mean you're on the right track. But how low can you go?

1 Lean against a wall, placing your feet about 1 foot away from the wall, and hold a medicine ball just below your chest, keeping your chin down.

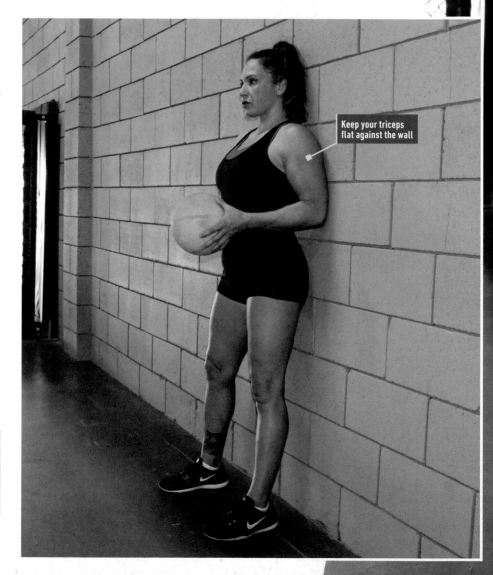

Keep your triceps flat against the wall

TIP
Keep a slight curve in your back to help you more easily slide down the wall.

Keep your head lifted and your chin down

2 Bend your knees to lower into a squat, with your legs at 90° angles, keeping the medicine ball close to your body. Reverse your movements to return to your starting position, then repeat this step for the duration listed in a workout.

MAKE IT **HARDER**

In step 2, hold the ball straight above your head, extending your arms fully.

BACKWARD OVERHEAD THROWS

Developing core strength helps you maintain energy and speed in your daily activities. Going from a curled squat to a fully extended leap can test the extremes of your body's capabilities. (And yelling *is* helpful!)

1 Stand with your feet hip-width apart, and hold a medicine ball in your hands between your legs. Bend at your hips, squat, and load your legs for the takeoff and extension.

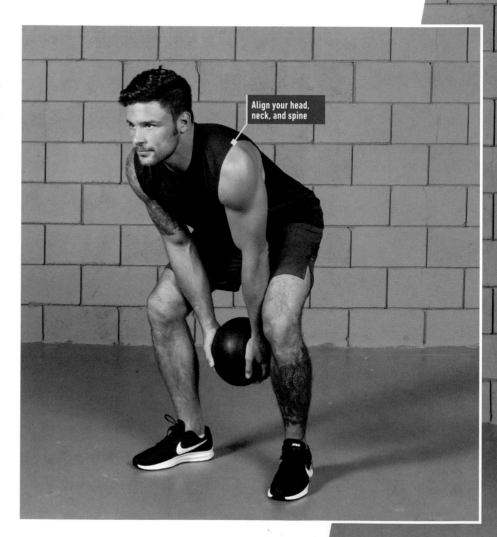

Align your head, neck, and spine

2 Throw your arms and head back and release the medicine ball backward as high and as far as possible while also jumping into the air. Pick up the ball and return to your starting position, then repeat these steps for the duration listed in a workout.

MAKE IT HARDER

In step 1, perform a burpee before continuing with step 2.

Push through your feet to help you jump off the ground

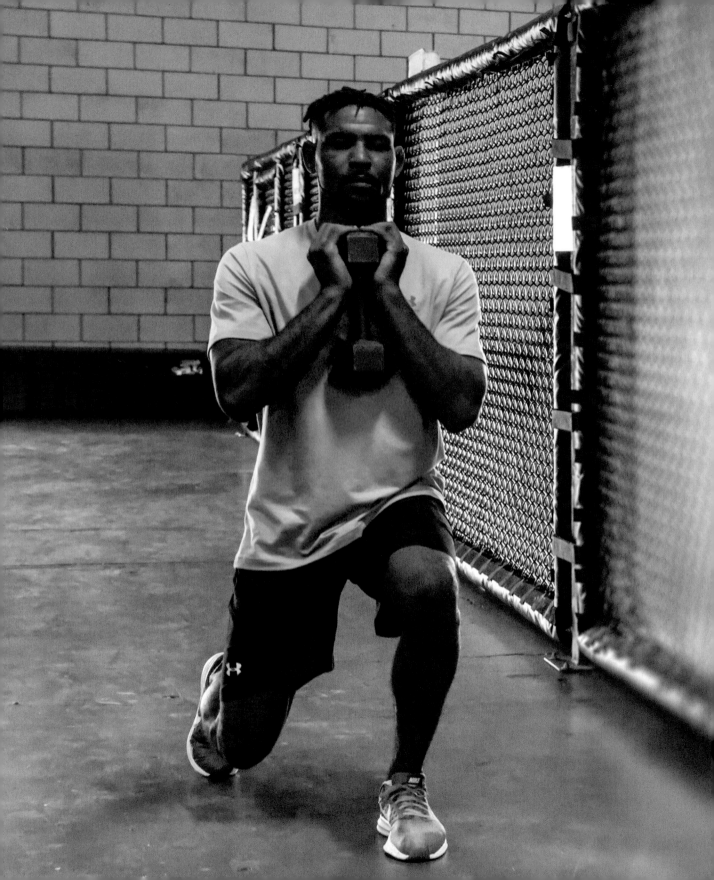

LOWER-BODY EXERCISES

PUSH KICKS

While a push kick is typically intended for a disciplinary defense or offense, the anatomy helps create balance and dexterity. Using your stability, this strike strengthens the abs, quads, calves, and mobility for major joints.

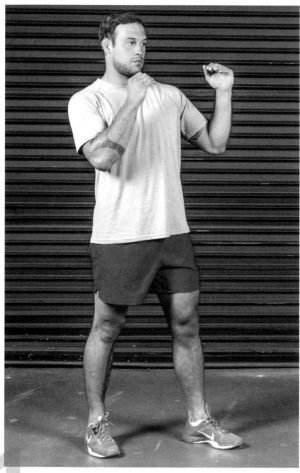

1 Stand with your feet hip-width apart, place your left leg slightly in front of your right leg, and place your slightly balled hands just under your chin.

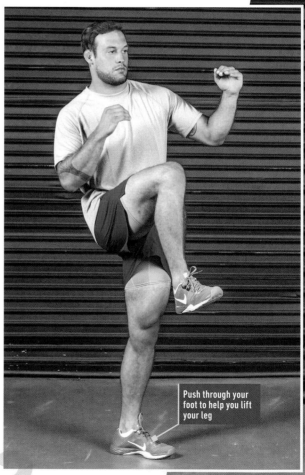

Push through your foot to help you lift your leg

2 Bend your right knee and begin to raise your right leg toward your chest.

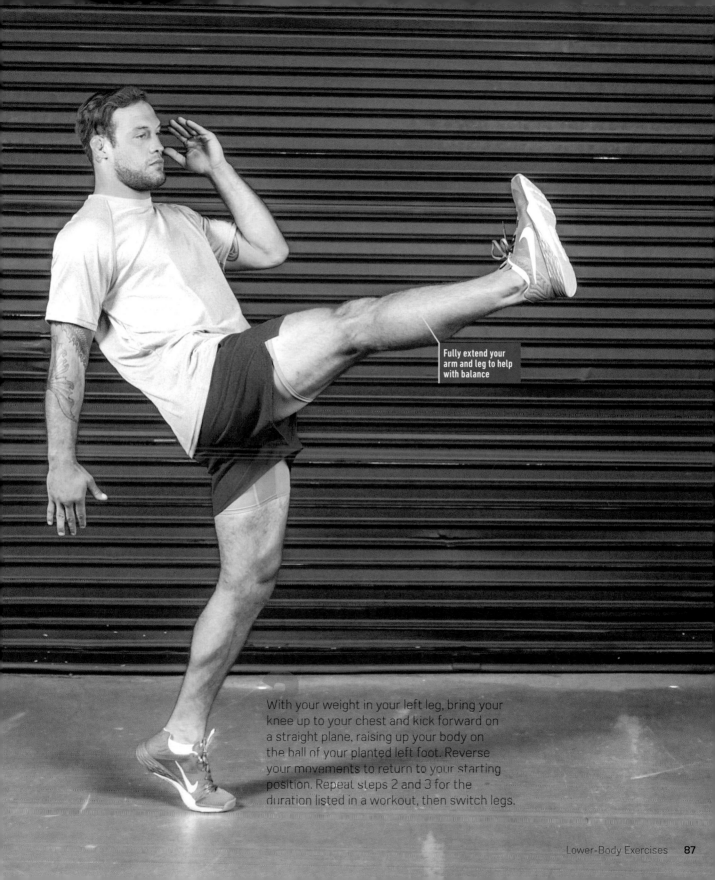

Fully extend your arm and leg to help with balance

With your weight in your left leg, bring your knee up to your chest and kick forward on a straight plane, raising up your body on the ball of your planted left foot. Reverse your movements to return to your starting position. Repeat steps 2 and 3 for the duration listed in a workout, then switch legs.

MEDICINE BALL JUMPS

Jumping over an obstacle can help you increase your speed, agility, endurance, coordination, and strength. The faster you go, the more demanding this exercise becomes—and the stronger the overall benefits.

1

Place a medicine ball on the ground, then stand next to the ball so it's at your right side. Slightly bend your knees to lower yourself into a semi-squat position, swinging your arms behind you.

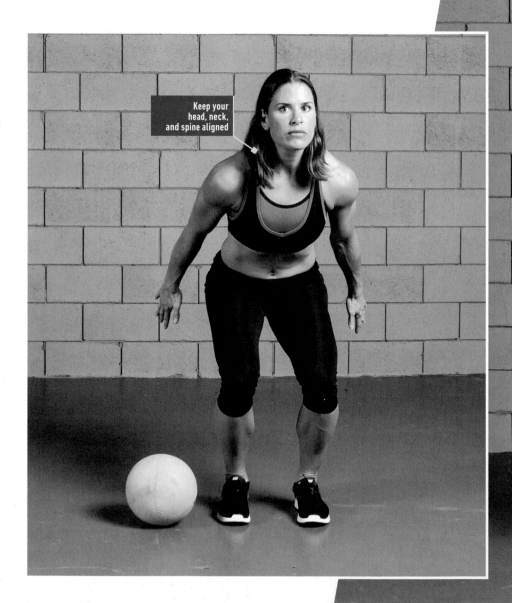

Keep your head, neck, and spine aligned

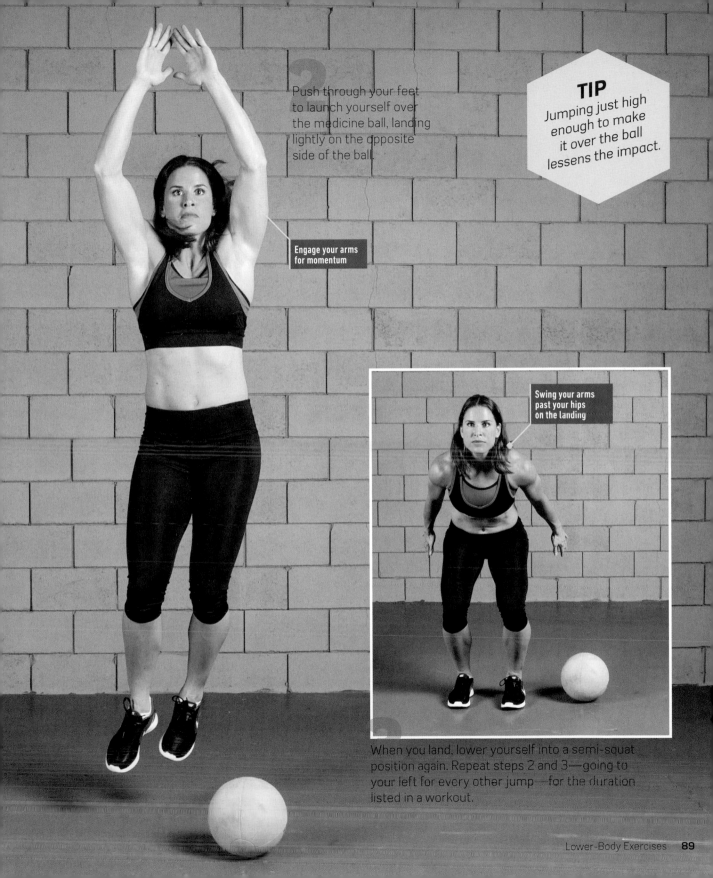

Push through your feet to launch yourself over the medicine ball, landing lightly on the opposite side of the ball.

Engage your arms for momentum

TIP
Jumping just high enough to make it over the ball lessens the impact.

Swing your arms past your hips on the landing

When you land, lower yourself into a semi-squat position again. Repeat steps 2 and 3—going to your left for every other jump—for the duration listed in a workout.

SIDE-TO-SIDE SHUFFLE

In MMA, this side-to-side motion serves as a way to be elusive and to cover as much lateral distance as possible in a short amount of time. Practicing this often and switching directions challenge your cardio and agility.

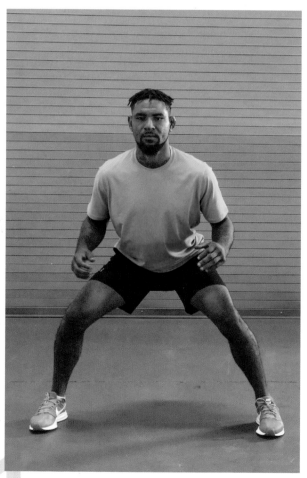

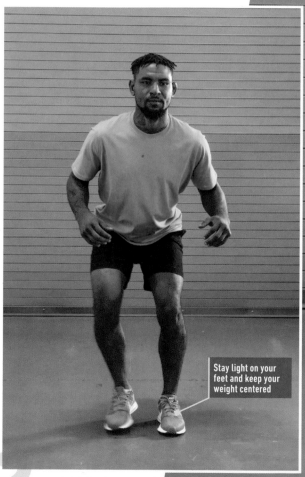

Stay light on your feet and keep your weight centered

Stand with your feet wider than hip-width apart and slightly bend your elbows to hold your hands near chest level, keeping your hips low.

Step your right foot to your left, engaging your arms as you move.

Keep your shoulders back and your chin down

Step your left foot to your left, continuing to engage your arms as you move. Repeat steps 2 and 3 for the duration listed in a workout, then reverse directions.

MAKE IT HARDER

In steps 2 and 3, perform punches, keeping your hands up in front of your face, as if blocking.

SIDE KICKS

Keep your hips, obliques, abs, and quads strong by keeping your posture and form true. These kicks are an agile but fun way to express MMA confidence while creating a flexion that builds and trims for lean muscle.

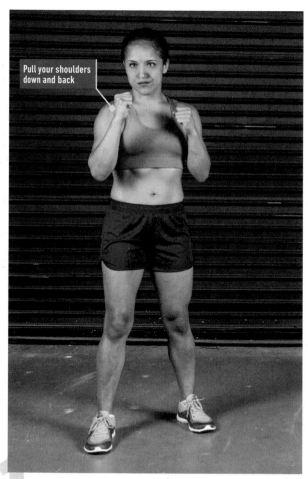

Pull your shoulders down and back

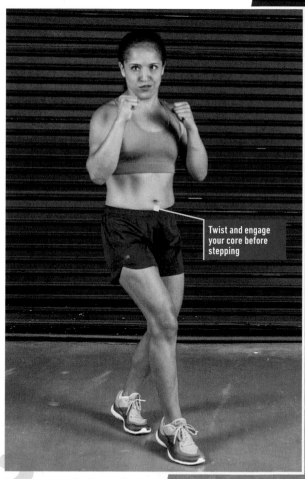

Twist and engage your core before stepping

1 Stand with your feet hip-width apart, place your right leg slightly in front of your left leg, and place your balled hands just under your chin.

2 Step your right foot across your body to directly in front of your left foot, bending your right knee as you prepare to kick.

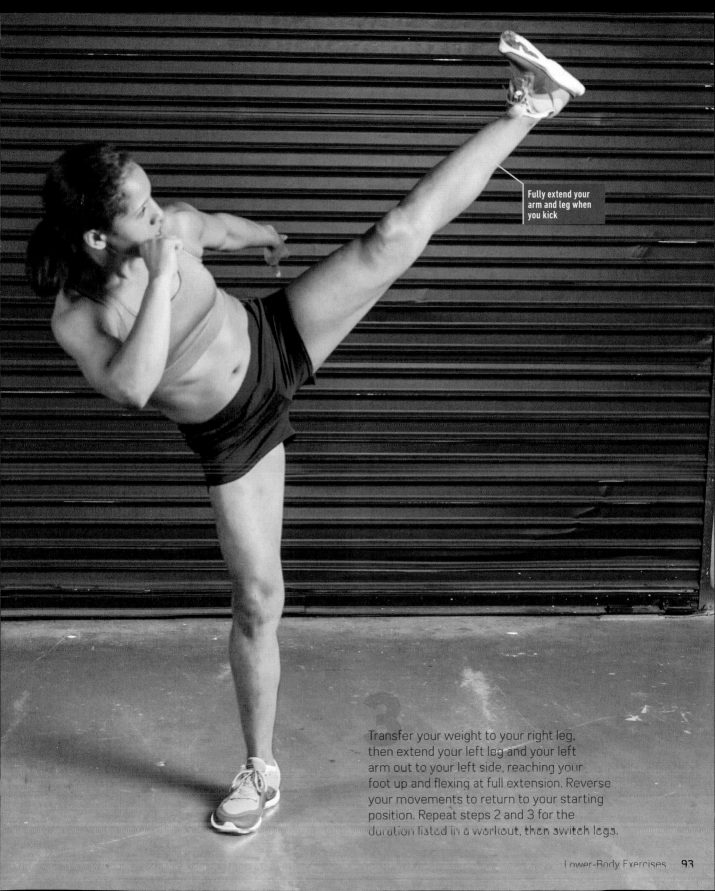

Fully extend your arm and leg when you kick

Transfer your weight to your right leg, then extend your left leg and your left arm out to your left side, reaching your foot up and flexing at full extension. Reverse your movements to return to your starting position. Repeat steps 2 and 3 for the duration listed in a workout, then switch legs.

PLATFORM STEP-UPS

For toning and strengthening leg muscles, few exercises work better than this one. Not only do you get the benefits of a one-legged squat, but you also get the fun and extension of throwing a Muay Thai kick at the top!

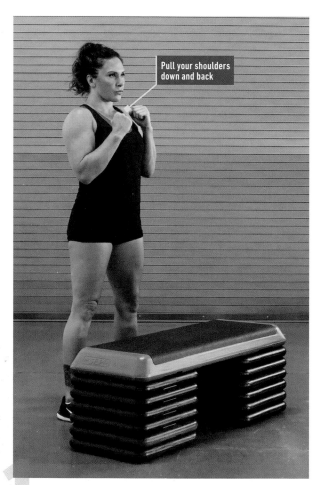

Pull your shoulders down and back

Place a step platform on the floor, elevate it to almost 2 feet, and stand facing the platform, keeping your balled hands near your face.

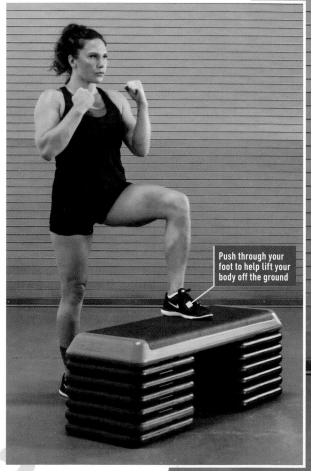

Push through your foot to help lift your body off the ground

Step your left foot on the platform and shift your weight forward to begin to bring yourself up onto the platform.

Keep your arms close to your body

TIP
The higher your step platform, the stronger your legs can become.

Lift your right leg off the ground, keeping it off the platform, and raise your knee to its highest point. Reverse your movements to return to your starting position. Repeat steps 2 and 3 for the duration listed in a workout, then switch legs.

MAKE IT HARDER

In step 1, hold a dumbbell in each hand, then perform steps 2 and 3.

MEDICINE BALL SQUATS

Squats replicate many everyday activities (like properly lifting and carrying). Holding a medicine ball can give your arms a burn, and the extra weight contributes to the power and conditioning distributed through the legs.

1 Stand with your feet hip-width apart, holding a stability ball at your chest with your hands.

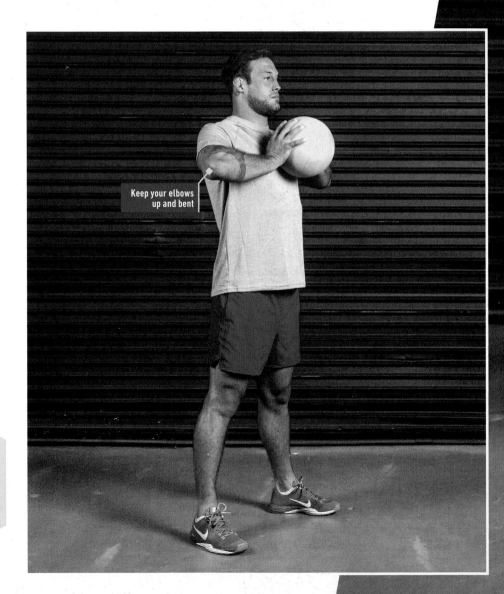

Keep your elbows up and bent

TIP
Engaging your core is additional conditioning and endurance building.

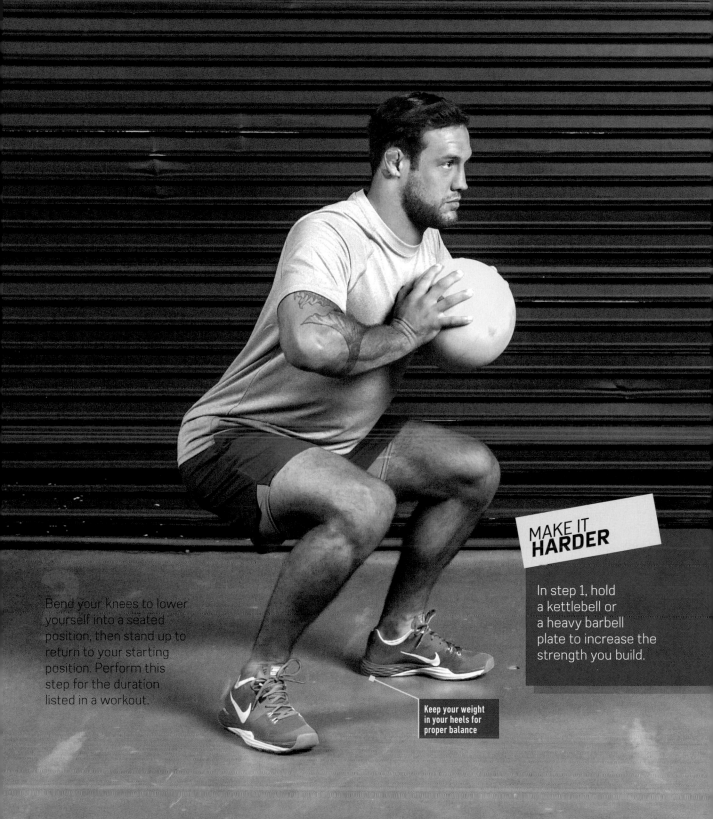

Bend your knees to lower yourself into a seated position, then stand up to return to your starting position. Perform this step for the duration listed in a workout.

MAKE IT **HARDER**

In step 1, hold a kettlebell or a heavy barbell plate to increase the strength you build.

Keep your weight in your heels for proper balance

SQUAT JUMPS

Jump squats are more dynamic than regular squats, helping to tone and shape calves, glutes, and quads. Jumping also challenges your cardiovascular system and improves your vertical agility and coordination.

1 Stand with your feet hip-width apart, slightly bend your knees to lower into a semi-squat, and relax your arms at your sides, slightly pulling them past your hips.

TIP
A proper squat jump landing is soft and silent.

Push through your feet to help you jump

2 Push through your feet and swing your arms forward and up as you jump straight up, fully extending your arms above your head, then try to softly land in your starting position. Repeat steps 2 and 3 for the duration listed in a workout.

Keep your hips forward when jumping

MAKE IT HARDER

In step 1, hold cables attached to a pulley system to increase your traction.

RUNNING BACKWARD

Running backward uses the opposite muscles used in running forward, changing things up and creating resistance. Going backward requires more effort, burning more calories and heightening our senses.

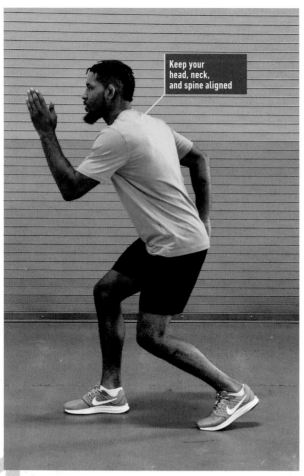

Keep your head, neck, and spine aligned

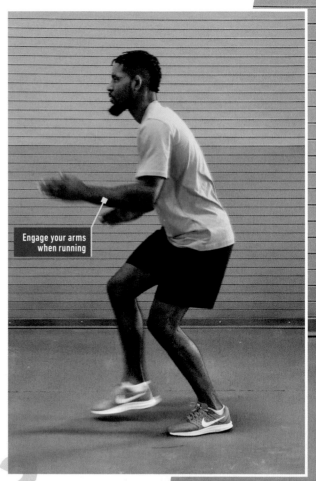

Engage your arms when running

1 Stand with your legs hip-width apart, putting your right leg in front and your left leg behind.

2 Quickly step your right leg behind you, putting the ball of your right foot on the ground before putting the heel of your right foot on the ground, keeping your right foot flat before taking the next step.

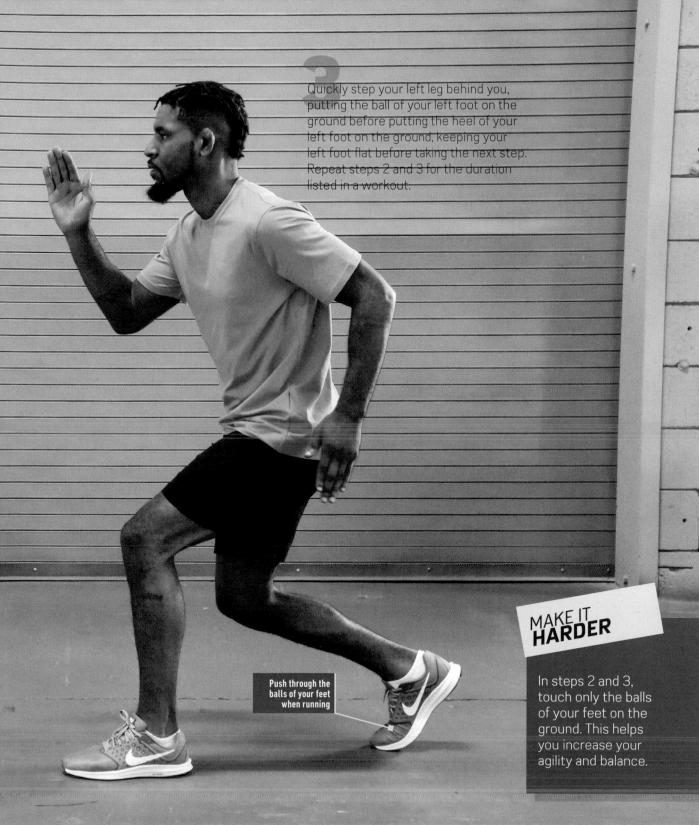

3

Quickly step your left leg behind you, putting the ball of your left foot on the ground before putting the heel of your left foot on the ground, keeping your left foot flat before taking the next step. Repeat steps 2 and 3 for the duration listed in a workout.

Push through the balls of your feet when running

MAKE IT **HARDER**

In steps 2 and 3, touch only the balls of your feet on the ground. This helps you increase your agility and balance.

TARGETS /// glutes, quads, calves, and hamstrings
EQUIPMENT /// none

BACKWARD LUNGES

This exercise demands you keep your weight in your forward leg, then you'll quickly change your pace with an aggressive push. Focus on form because you're taking an explosive backward action with a forward attitude.

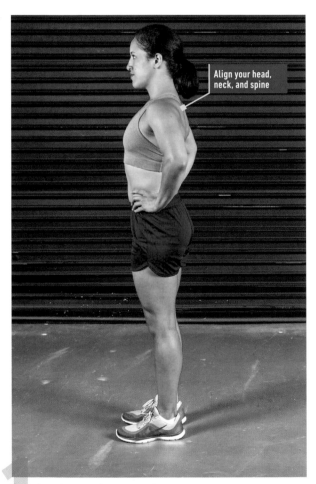

Align your head, neck, and spine

1 Stand with your feet together and your hands on your hips.

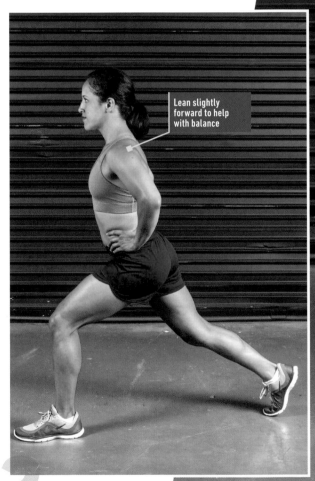

Lean slightly forward to help with balance

2 Step your right foot backward, slightly bending your right knee and balancing your right leg on the tip of your toes, and bend your left knee as you begin to lower yourself to the ground.

TIP

The slower you lunge and the faster you push, the more you'll burn.

MAKE IT HARDER

In step 1, hold dumbbells in your hands. In steps 2 and 3, swing your arms overhead as you lunge.

Form 90° angles with your legs

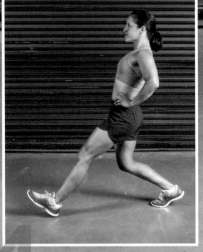

Lower yourself until your left knee forms a 90° angle and your right knee almost touches the ground. Start to shift your weight from your front leg to your back leg.

Explosively push through your left foot to force yourself back to your starting position. Repeat steps 2 to 4 for the duration listed in a workout, then switch legs.

TARGETS /// hamstrings and core
EQUIPMENT /// none

SQUAT STEPS

Keeping a healthy musculoskeletal system is crucial to successful training. These squats can help with that, including being essential for performing functional and strengthening movements with your lower body and joints.

1

Stand with your feet hip-width apart and bend your elbows to form 45° angles with your arms, then squat down, keeping your weight in your heels and your knees and hips hinged.

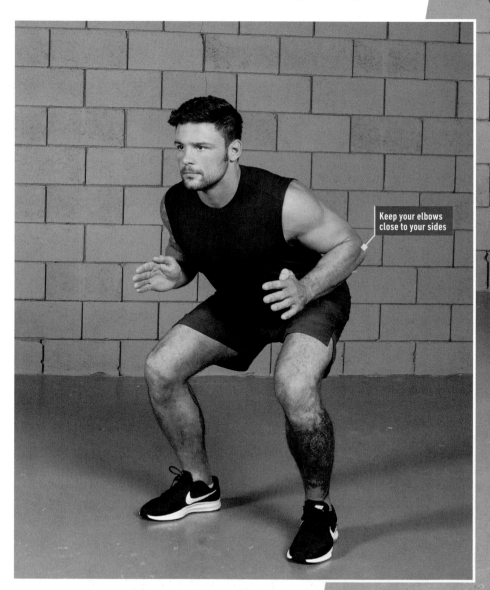

Keep your elbows close to your sides

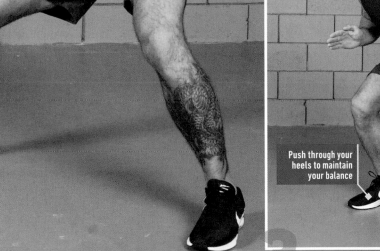

Keep your head on the same plane

MAKE IT HARDER

In step 1, hold a medicine ball in your hands at your chest.

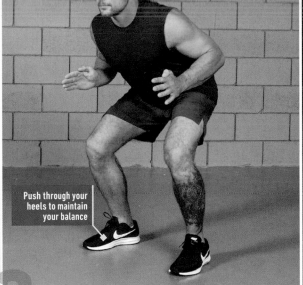

Push through your heels to maintain your balance

Step your right foot to the right, continuing to maintain your squatting position.

Step your left foot toward your right foot to return to your starting position. Repeat this step for the duration listed in a workout, then reverse your direction.

BACKWARD SQUAT STEPS

Squats are an excellent exercise for enhancing ankle mobility, leg endurance, and overall balance—an ideal addition to any workout—and when done in reverse, they can further strengthen your core stability.

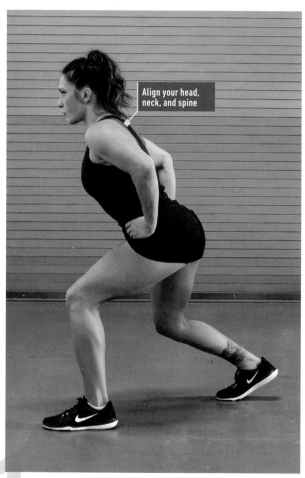

Stand with your feet hip-width apart, putting your left foot in front of your right foot and bending your right knee to keep your head over your toes.

Align your head, neck, and spine

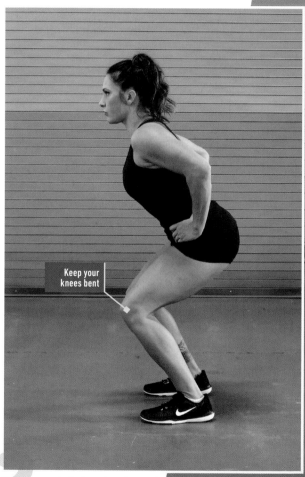

Step your left foot back until it's parallel with your right foot, keeping your hips back, your knees hinged, and your back engaged, and maintain your balance by keeping your weight in your heels.

Keep your knees bent

In step 1, hold dumbbells or a resistance band in your hands to increase resistance, then perform steps 2 and 3.

Shift through the balls of your feet to help with balance

Step your left foot backward, then step your right foot backward until it's parallel with your left foot. Perform steps 2 and 3 for the duration listed in a workout.

JUMPING KNEES

Athletically, taking flight has many benefits. This exercise uses your core for pull and explosion; legs for endurance and height; and arms for momentum and balance.

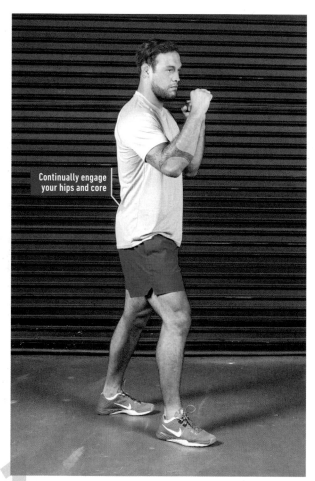

Continually engage your hips and core

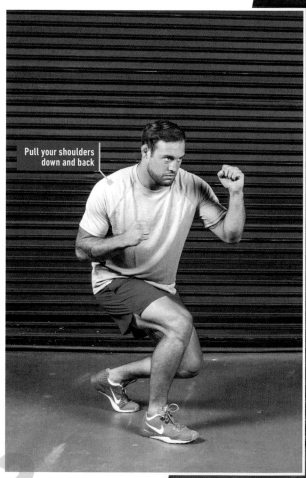

Pull your shoulders down and back

1 Stand with your feet hip-width apart, placing your right leg in front of your left leg, and hold your hands near your face.

2 Squat down until your right knee is at a 90° angle, with your left leg serving as a support, then swing your arms up as you spring your body upward.

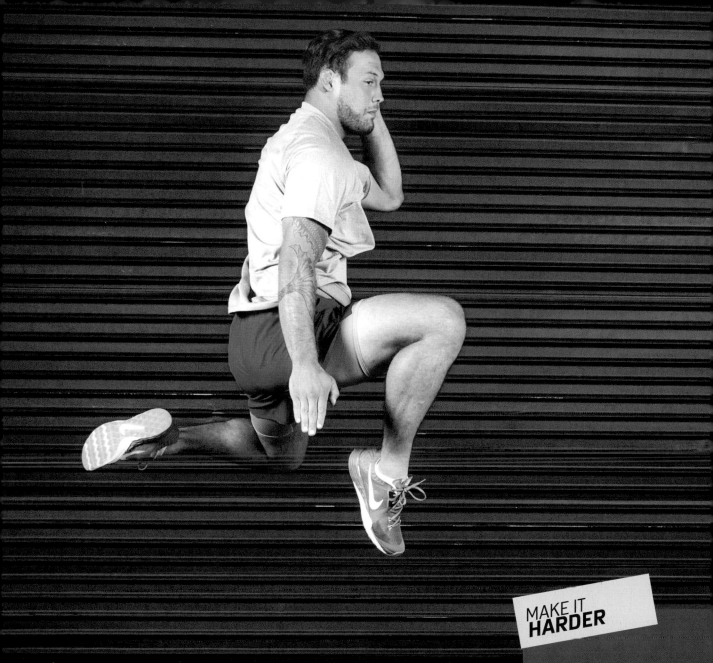

MAKE IT
HARDER

In step 1, start by
grabbing a pullup bar.
In step 2, bring your
bent knees toward
your bent elbows.

Push your left foot into the ground, lifting your body
off the ground and pointing your toe down for
maximum flexion, and bring your right knee toward
your chest. Once you land, return to your starting
position. Repeat steps 2 and 3 for the duration listed
in a workout, then switch legs.

TARGETS /// quads, calves, shins, glutes, lower back, hamstrings, and thighs
EQUIPMENT /// none

HEEL-TO-TOE ROCKERS & SQUATS

Warming up can help activate muscles and blood flow. Rockers create a fluid motion from front to back and top to bottom, lightly challenging the smaller muscles of your legs and preparing the major muscles to do work.

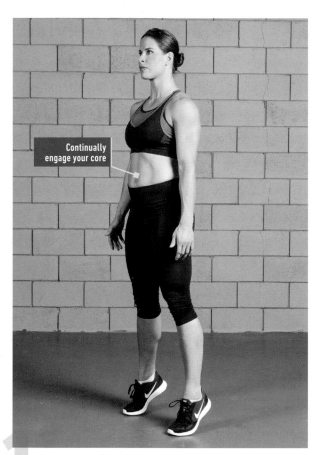

Continually engage your core

Stand with your feet hip-width apart, relax your arms at your sides, and roll your weight onto the tips of your toes.

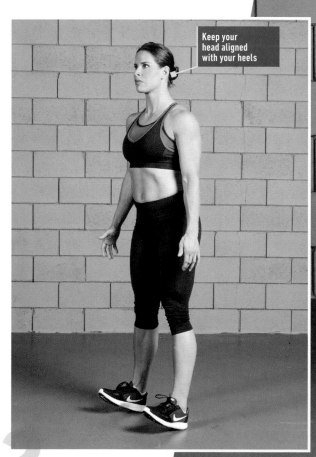

Keep your head aligned with your heels

Rock backward to put your heels on the ground and lift your toes off the ground.

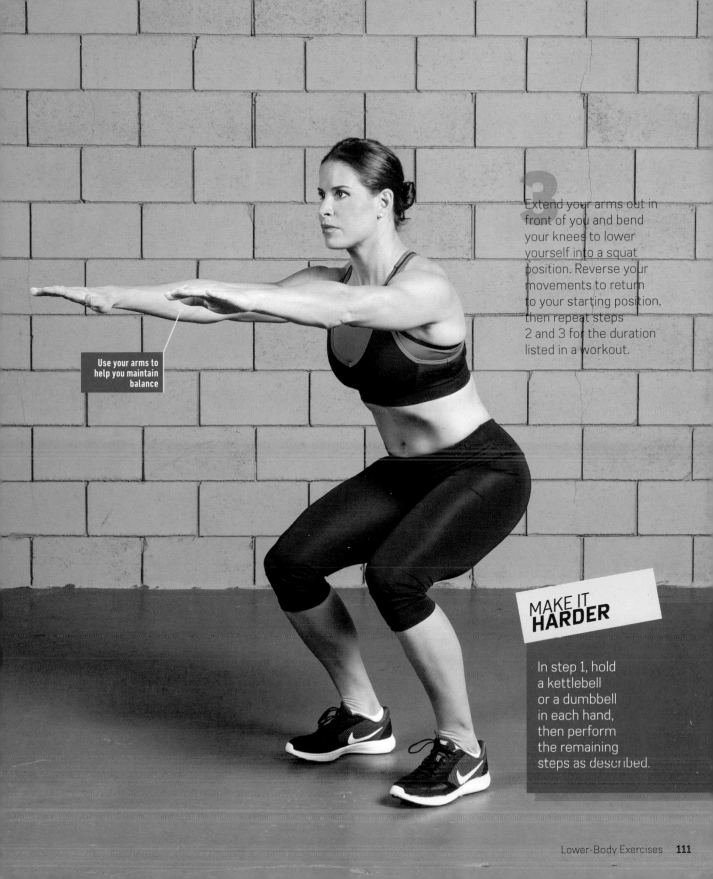

3 Extend your arms out in front of you and bend your knees to lower yourself into a squat position. Reverse your movements to return to your starting position, then repeat steps 2 and 3 for the duration listed in a workout.

Use your arms to help you maintain balance

MAKE IT
HARDER

In step 1, hold a kettlebell or a dumbbell in each hand, then perform the remaining steps as described.

SINGLE-LEG SQUATS

Not only does this exercise increase your explosiveness and power, but it also enhances endurance. These improvements can help you with your balance while targeting individually allows for equal strengthening.

1 Stand in front of a step platform with your feet hip-width apart, holding a dumbbell in each hand with an overhand grip. Relax your hands at your sides, then bend your right knee to place the front of your right foot on the platform behind you.

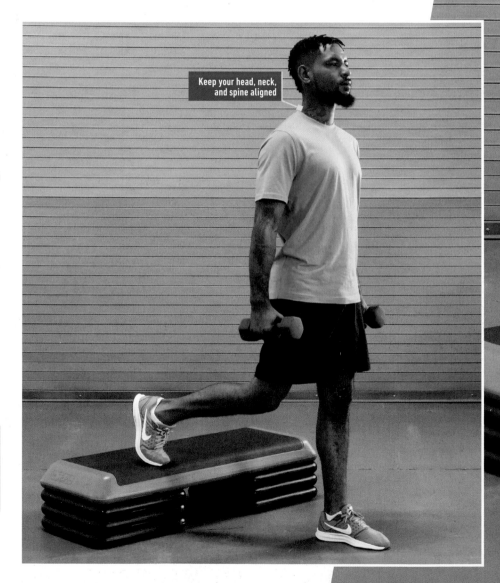

Keep your head, neck, and spine aligned

TIP
Being mindful of your technique can help prevent any injuries.

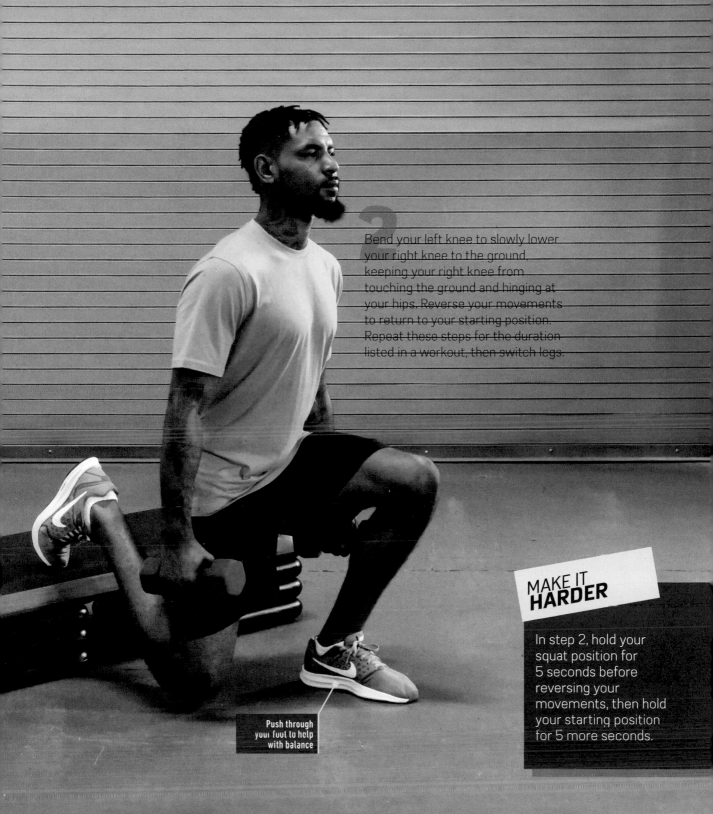

Bend your left knee to slowly lower your right knee to the ground, keeping your right knee from touching the ground and hinging at your hips. Reverse your movements to return to your starting position. Repeat these steps for the duration listed in a workout, then switch legs.

Push through your foot to help with balance

MAKE IT **HARDER**

In step 2, hold your squat position for 5 seconds before reversing your movements, then hold your starting position for 5 more seconds.

SINGLE-HIP THRUSTS

Keeping your hips up and independently working your flexed legs can increase your endurance. Dropping your hips and rocking engages abs, hamstrings, and glutes, strengthening vital muscles for an MMA physique.

1 Rest your weight across your shoulders on the elevated step platform, extending your arms out to your sides. Bend your knees at 90° angles, and keep your feet flat on the ground and your body parallel with the ground.

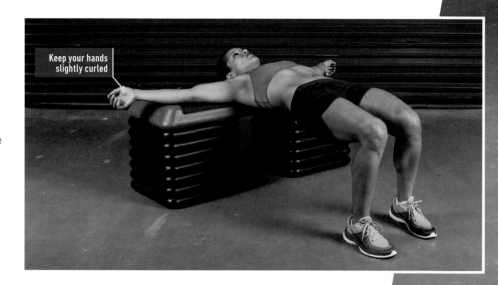

Keep your hands slightly curled

2 Lift your left leg off the ground to fully extend that leg away from your body, engaging your glutes and abs, then lift up at the hips.

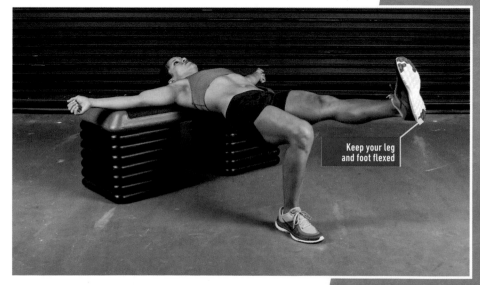

Keep your leg and foot flexed

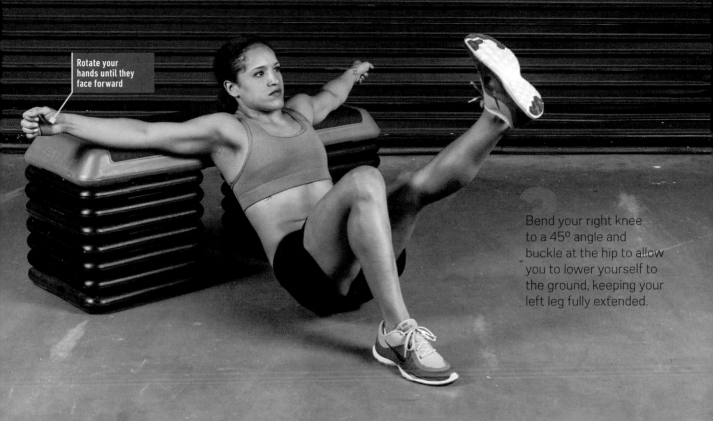

Rotate your
hands until they
face forward

Bend your right knee
to a 45° angle and
buckle at the hip to allow
you to lower yourself to
the ground, keeping your
left leg fully extended.

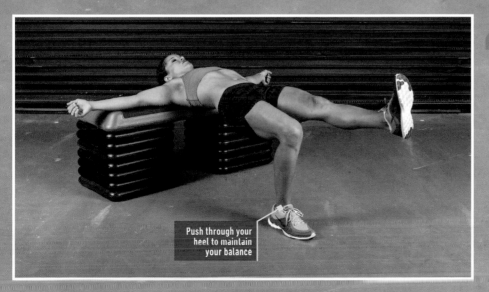

Push through your
heel to maintain
your balance

Press through your right
foot to lift yourself back
up until your body is again
parallel with the ground,
leading with the hips and
continuing to keep your
left leg extended and
your left foot flexed,
then return your left leg
to its starting position.
Repeat steps 2 through 4
for the duration listed in
a workout, then switch legs.

TARGETS /// quads, legs, hamstrings, adductors, and hip flexors
EQUIPMENT /// soccer ball (or a medicine ball)

SOCCER BALL TOUCHES

Shifting, jumping, and balancing while incorporating these ball touches takes concentration and dexterity. Focus and cardio can improve immensely as you commit to moving and understanding your body mechanics.

1

Place a soccer ball on the ground and stand just behind the ball, placing your feet hip-width apart. Bend your right knee to quickly tap your right foot on top of the ball.

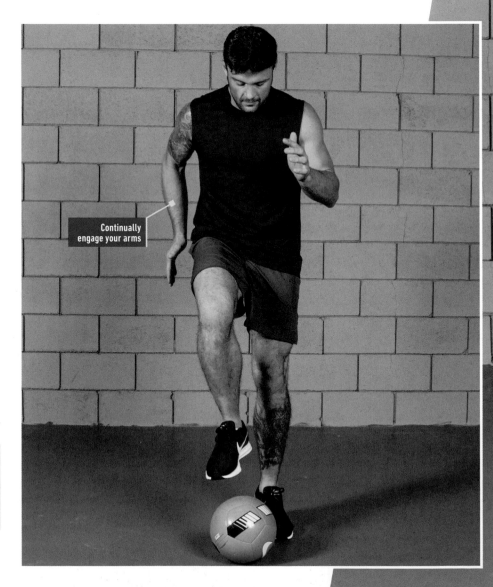

Continually engage your arms

TIP
Look at the ball, but stay focused on form and being light on your feet.

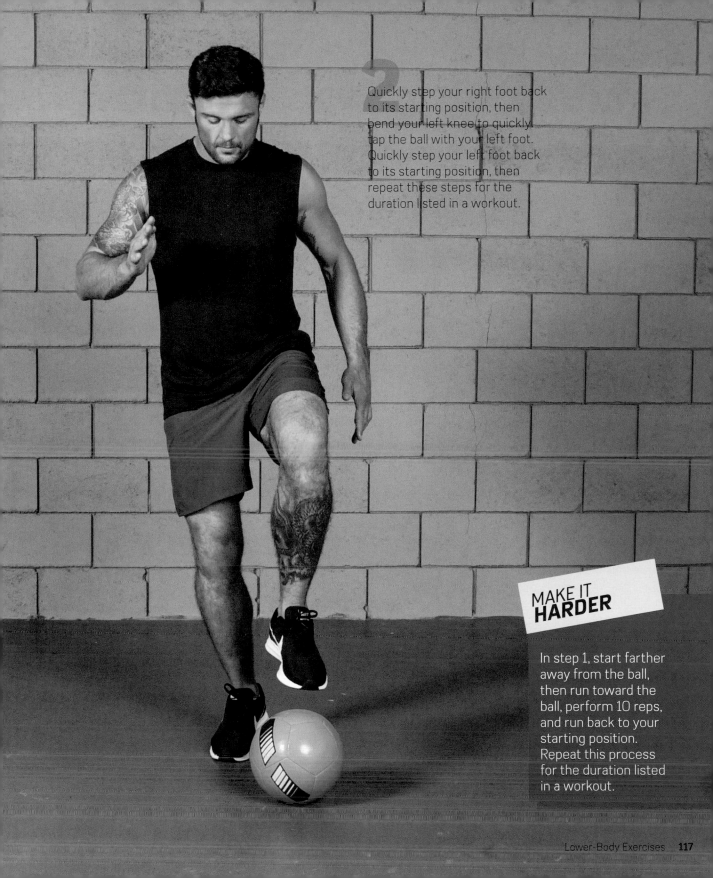

2 Quickly step your right foot back to its starting position, then bend your left knee to quickly tap the ball with your left foot. Quickly step your left foot back to its starting position, then repeat these steps for the duration listed in a workout.

MAKE IT **HARDER**

In step 1, start farther away from the ball, then run toward the ball, perform 10 reps, and run back to your starting position. Repeat this process for the duration listed in a workout.

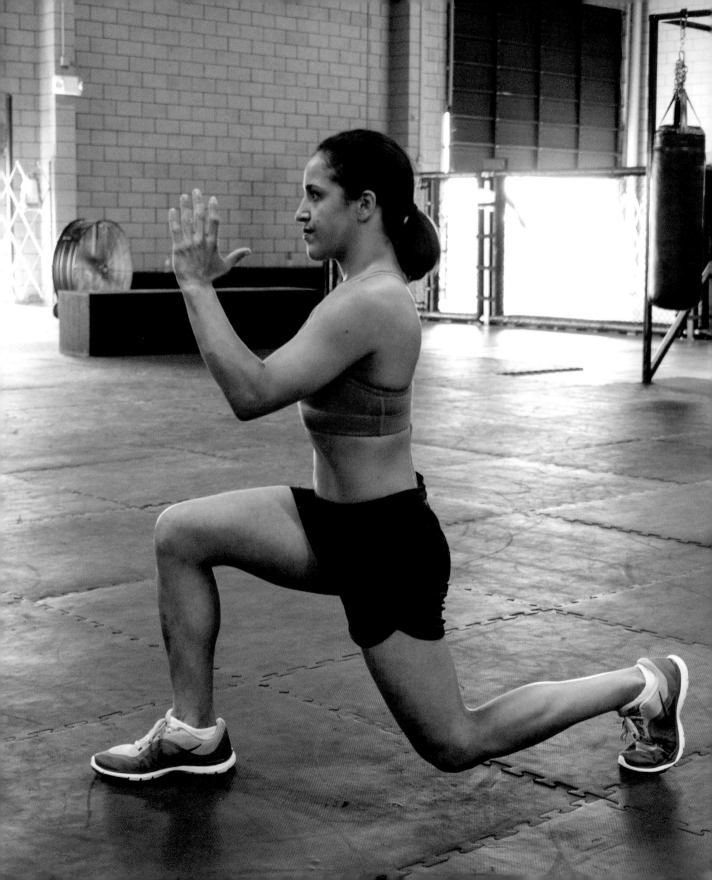

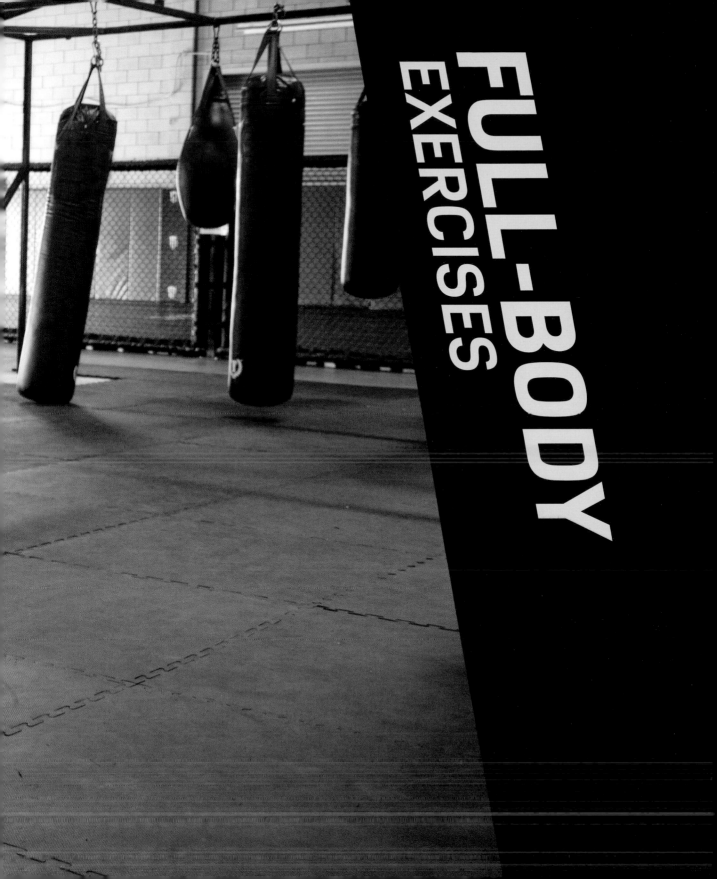

FULL-BODY
EXERCISES

TARGETS /// arms, legs, and abs
EQUIPMENT /// none

SHADOW BOXING

Perhaps the toughest battle you'll ever fight is the one within yourself. Use your cardio, flexibility, technique, and drive to improve your confidence—and let your creativity flow.

1 Stand in an area free from any obstacles, keeping your feet hip-width apart, then stand in a fight stance. (See pages 16–21 for examples of stances.).

2 Perform jabs, crosses, hooks, elbows, knees, and kicks. (See pages 16–21 for examples.) Switch your feet and your arms and legs as you rotate from move to move. Repeat this step for the duration listed in a workout.

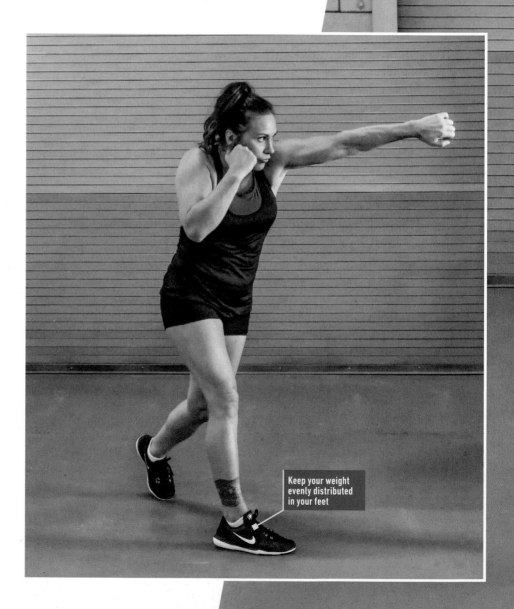

Keep your weight evenly distributed in your feet

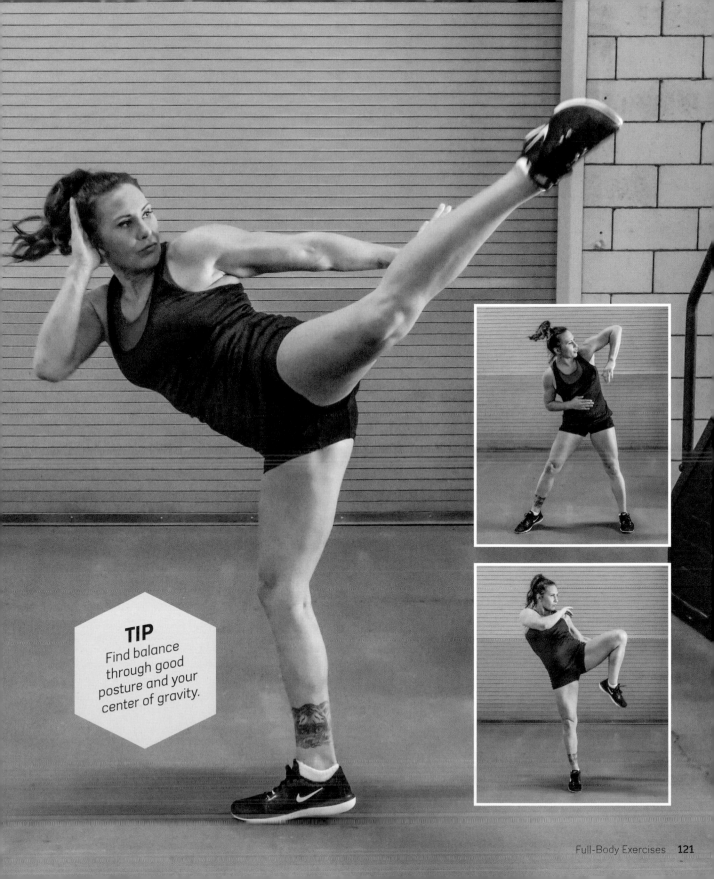

TIP
Find balance through good posture and your center of gravity.

TARGETS /// legs, glutes, arms, chest, back, shoulders, and core
EQUIPMENT /// medicine ball

MEDICINE BALL SQUAT TOSSES

This exercise focuses on functionality and practicality in developing fast twitch. It can also optimize reaction times while transferring energy from your lower body to your upper body, impacting every muscle group in these areas.

1 Stand with your feet hip-width apart, holding a medicine ball in your hands at your chest. Bend your knees to lower yourself into a squat position.

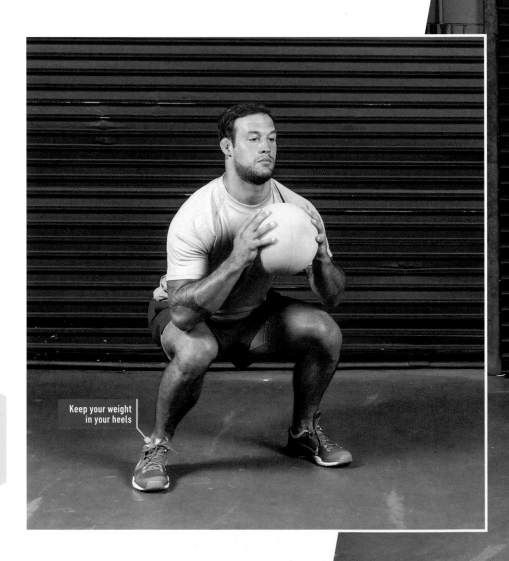

Keep your weight in your heels

TIP
Your elbows touching your knees is a good indicator that you're going low enough.

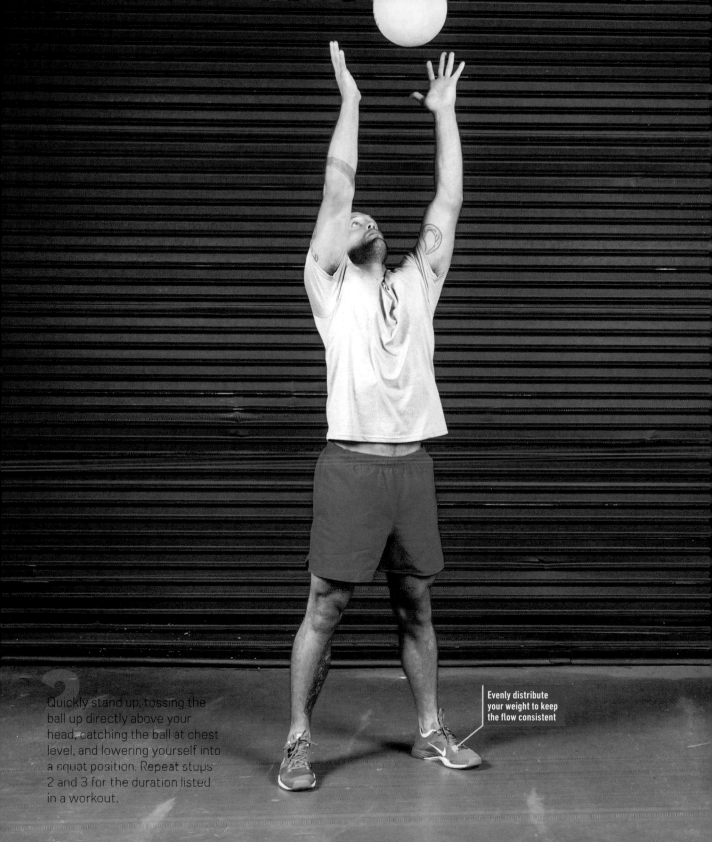

Quickly stand up, tossing the ball up directly above your head, catching the ball at chest level, and lowering yourself into a squat position. Repeat steps 2 and 3 for the duration listed in a workout.

Evenly distribute your weight to keep the flow consistent

LATERAL CRAWL

For this exercise, your engaged abs, tucked hips, and bent knees can help you maintain your balance and increase your core strength toward stability while simultaneously lifting the opposite hand and foot off the ground.

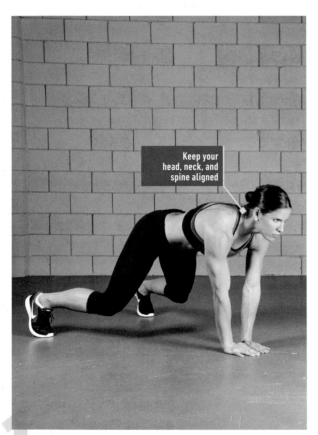

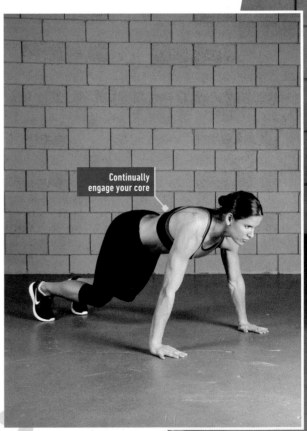

Keep your head, neck, and spine aligned

Continually engage your core

1 Place your hands side by side on the ground, pointing your fingers forward and slightly bending your elbows, then bend your knees, tuck your hips, and balance your weight on the balls of your feet, keeping your legs wider than hip-width apart.

2 Step your left hand and your right leg to the left, keeping your arms wider than shoulder-width apart and your feet close together.

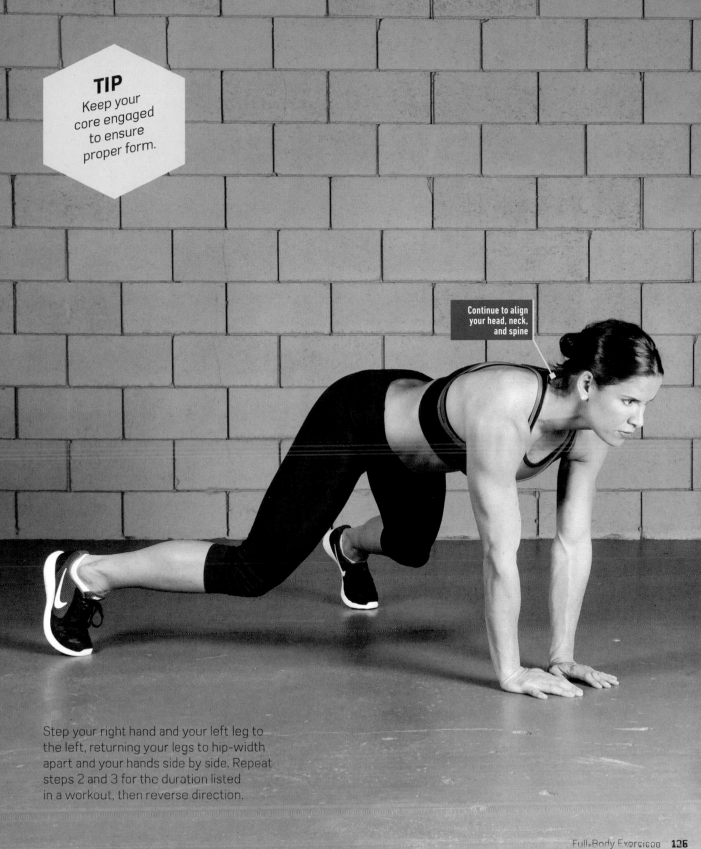

TIP
Keep your core engaged to ensure proper form.

Continue to align your head, neck, and spine

Step your right hand and your left leg to the left, returning your legs to hip-width apart and your hands side by side. Repeat steps 2 and 3 for the duration listed in a workout, then reverse direction.

HIGH SKIPS

Jumping benefits you in many ways: to get your heart rate up, to get your blood pumping, and to build a fast twitch in your agility muscles. On a deeper level, they make for a good time and teach us to be explosive in play.

1

Stand with your feet hip-width apart and your arms relaxed at your side, then start a skipping motion by raising your right knee and your left arm up as you push through your left foot to launch yourself off the ground.

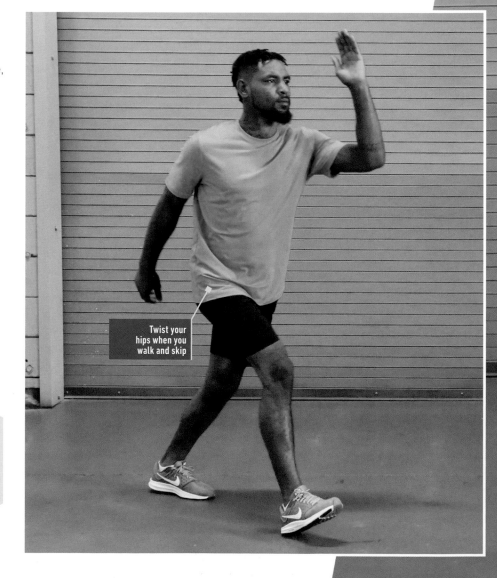

Twist your hips when you walk and skip

TIP
Pushing with momentum helps you learn to resist muscle fatigue.

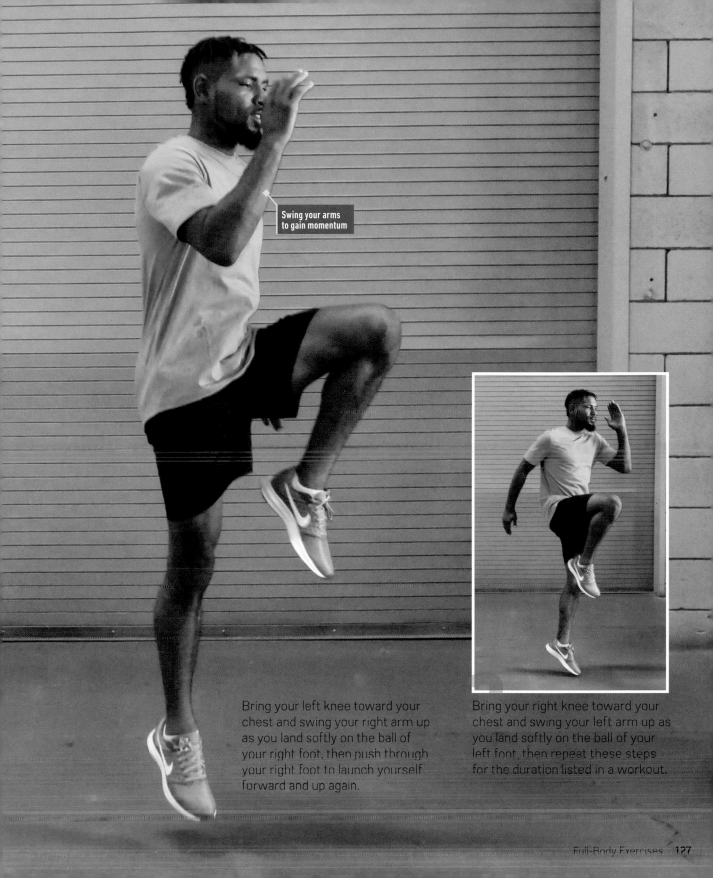

Swing your arms to gain momentum

Bring your left knee toward your chest and swing your right arm up as you land softly on the ball of your right foot, then push through your right foot to launch yourself forward and up again.

Bring your right knee toward your chest and swing your left arm up as you land softly on the ball of your left foot, then repeat these steps for the duration listed in a workout.

TARGETS /// shoulders, back, and arms
EQUIPMENT /// heavy bag

GROUND & POUND

This exercise is your chance to really let it all out and beat something up—rather than someone. Along with its mental and technical benefits, you'll also give your heart and lungs a workout—great for building endurance.

1 Place a heavy bag on the ground, put your left knee on the bag, and balance your left leg on the tips of your left foot, extending your right leg out to your right side and planting your right foot for balance. Place your left hand on the left side of the bag, then punch the bag with your right hand.

TIP
You can also sit on or straddle the heavy bag.

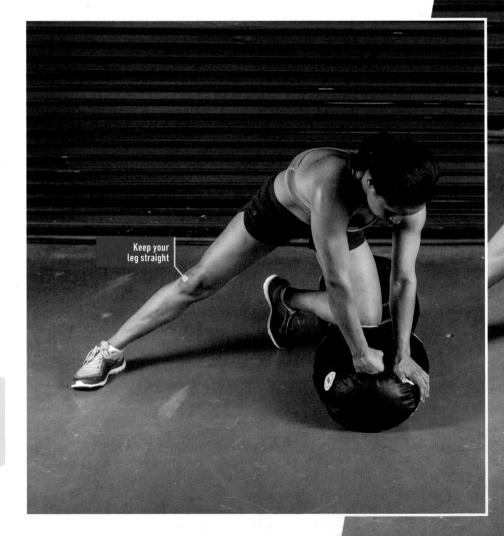

Keep your leg straight

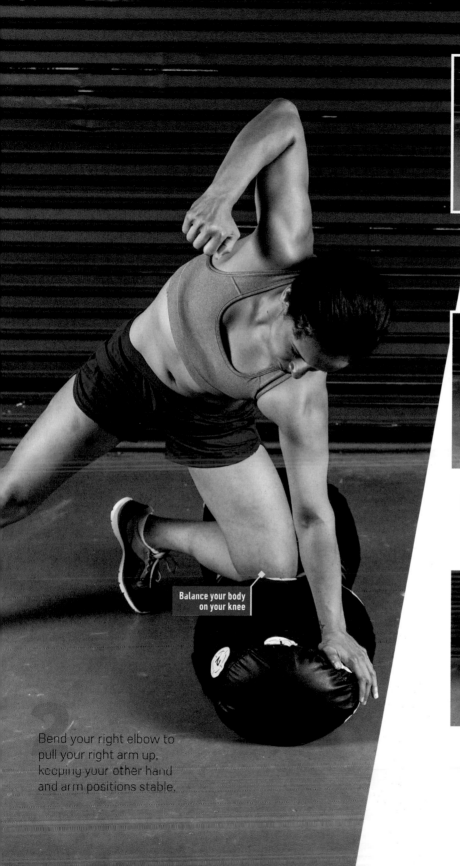

Balance your body on your knee

Bend your right elbow to pull your right arm up, keeping your other hand and arm positions stable.

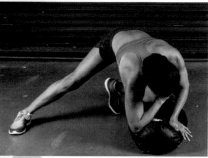

Quickly bring your right elbow down and into the right side of the bag.

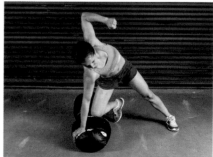

Replace your right elbow with your right hand and switch your left knee with your right knee, then jump to the other side of the bag.

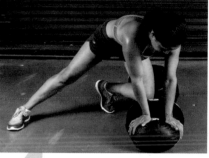

Push through your hands to launch yourself over the bag, then repeat steps 2 to 5 for the duration listed in a workout.

TARGETS /// quads, glutes, thighs, hamstrings, and calves
EQUIPMENT /// medicine ball

MEDICINE BALL LATERAL LUNGES

By lunging side to side, you increase the isometric advantages on each side of your body, creating optimal strength and range of motion. Form and technique can also help you sculpt your whole body evenly.

1

Stand with your feet wider than hip-width apart and hold a medicine ball in your hands at your chest.

Continually engage your core

TIP
Keep your weight in your heels and bend at your hips.

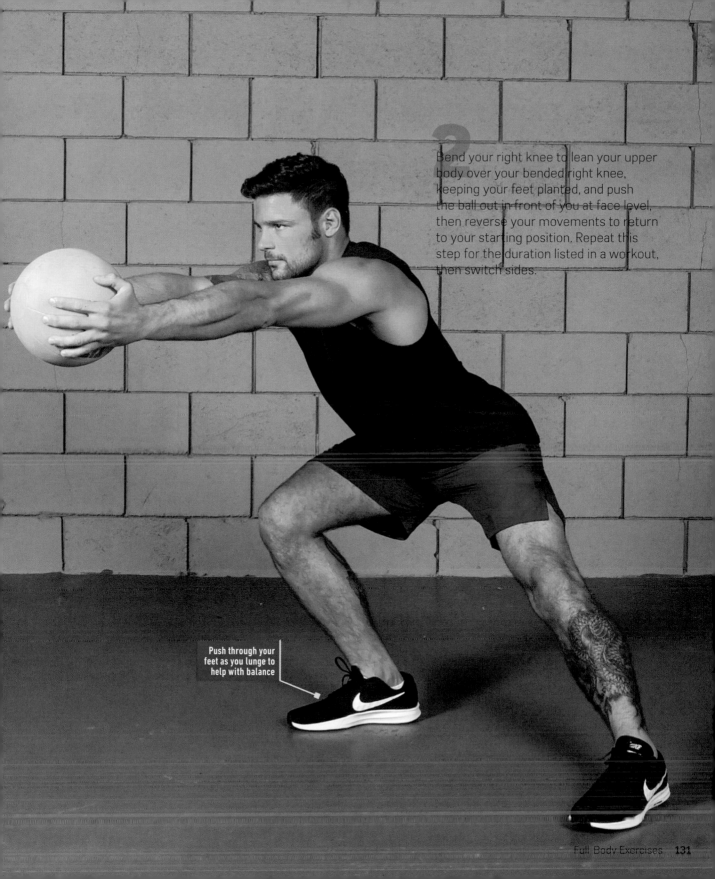

2 Bend your right knee to lean your upper body over your bended right knee, keeping your feet planted, and push the ball out in front of you at face level, then reverse your movements to return to your starting position. Repeat this step for the duration listed in a workout, then switch sides.

Push through your feet as you lunge to help with balance

TARGETS /// abs, glutes, quads, hamstrings, and calves
EQUIPMENT /// dumbbell

GOBLET CARRY

Using weights while performing a lunge makes your muscles, especially your abs, quads, and hamstrings, more dynamic, leading to more strength and lean muscle. This exercise also encourages the ability to stay balanced.

1

Stand with your feet hip-width apart and hold a dumbbell vertically at your chest between your palms, keeping your elbows tight to your core.

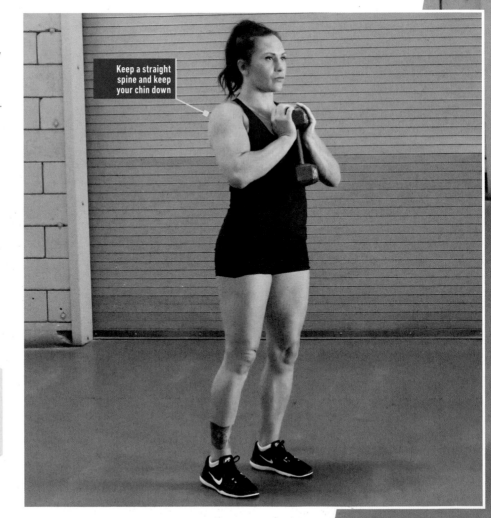

Keep a straight spine and keep your chin down

TIP
Step first, then lower your knee once you have balance.

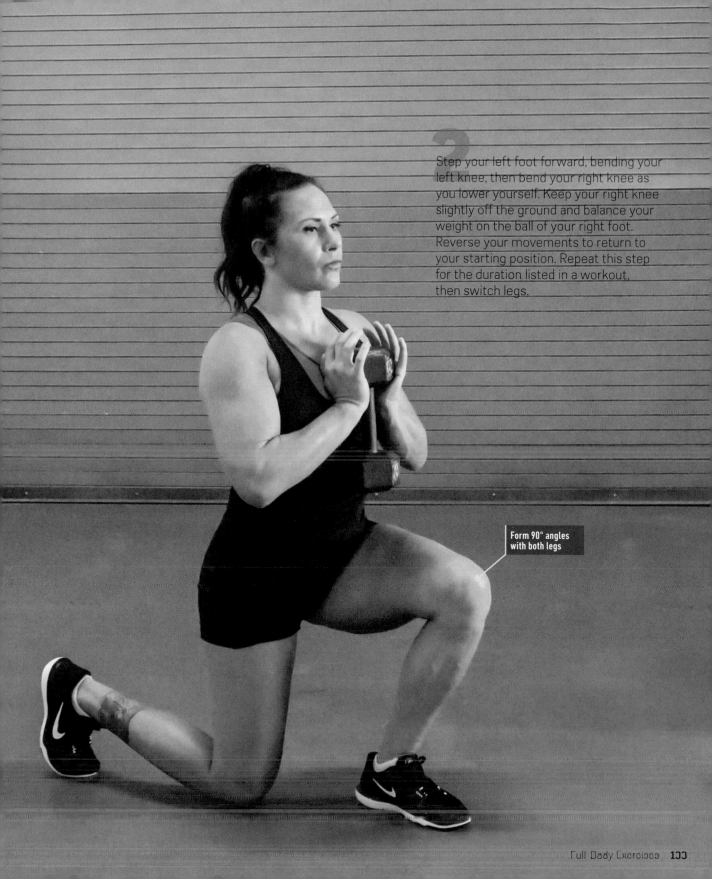

2 Step your left foot forward, bending your left knee, then bend your right knee as you lower yourself. Keep your right knee slightly off the ground and balance your weight on the ball of your right foot. Reverse your movements to return to your starting position. Repeat this step for the duration listed in a workout, then switch legs.

Form 90° angles with both legs

SIT-OUT ROTATION

Simultaneously engaging different muscle groups in an active rotation allows you to increase your flexibility, heart rate, and circulation. It also loosens the joints and intensely works each muscle in a cooperative effort.

1 Place your hands flat on the ground, pointing your fingers forward. Place your feet wider than hip-width apart, balancing your legs on the flexed balls of your feet

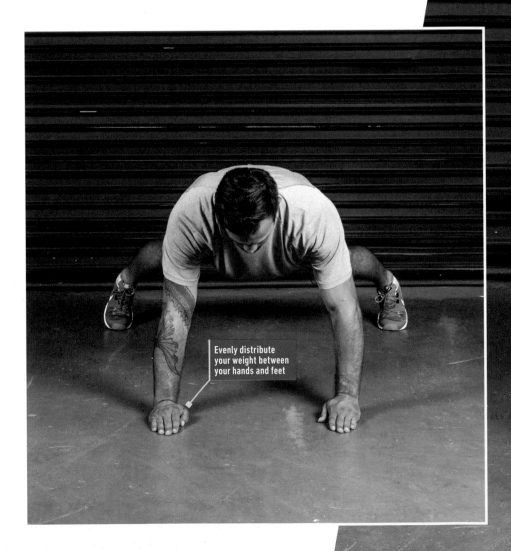

Evenly distribute your weight between your hands and feet

TIP

Shifting your weight before moving makes the rotation quicker.

Keep your palm open after twisting

Lift your right leg and left hand off the ground to twist your body to the left at your hips, keeping your left elbow tight to your body, then reverse your movements to return to your starting position. Repeat steps 2 and 3 for the duration listed in a workout, then switch sides.

TARGETS /// abs, obliques, and legs
EQUIPMENT /// none

PUSHUP ROTATION

This exercise creates a challenge to your balance as well as engages your core independently on each side. Turning at the top and diligent form make for an exceptional muscle-building, fat-burning performance enhancer.

1 Put your hands flat on the ground directly below your shoulders, pointing your fingers forward, and balance your weight evenly between your hands and the tips of your feet.

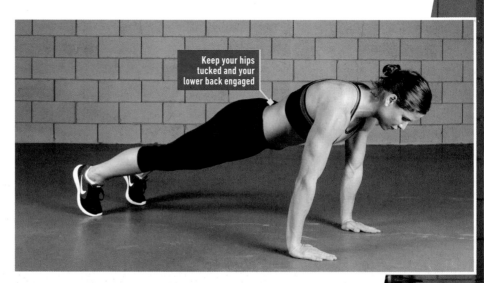

Keep your hips tucked and your lower back engaged

2 Bend your elbows to lower yourself toward the ground, keeping your chest lifted and your elbows tight to your sides.

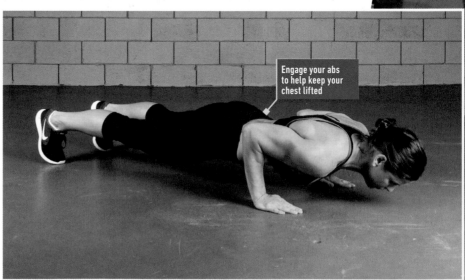

Engage your abs to help keep your chest lifted

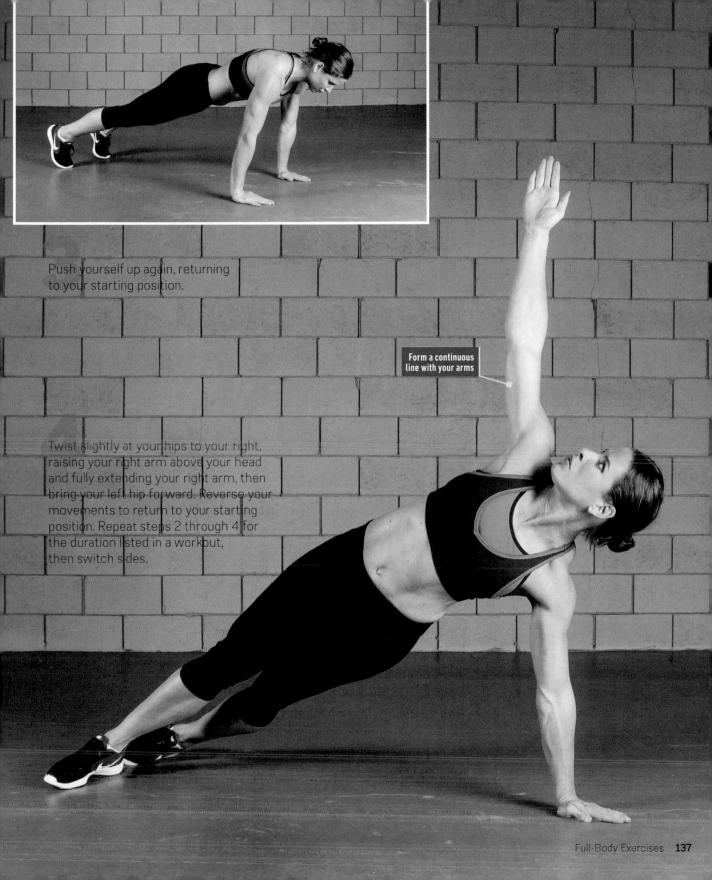

Push yourself up again, returning to your starting position.

Twist slightly at your hips to your right, raising your right arm above your head and fully extending your right arm, then bring your left hip forward. Reverse your movements to return to your starting position. Repeat steps 2 through 4 for the duration listed in a workout, then switch sides.

Form a continuous line with your arms

ONE-ARMED DUMBBELL ROW

Form is key with this multi-joint, multi-muscle exercise. Harnessing energy from the ground up affects many areas, including stamina, mobility, strength, and power.

1 Stand with your feet hip-width apart and your left foot 2 feet in front of your right foot, placing your left hand on your left knee to help bear some weight. Bend at your waist while keeping your back straight and hold a dumbbell in your right hand with an overhand grip.

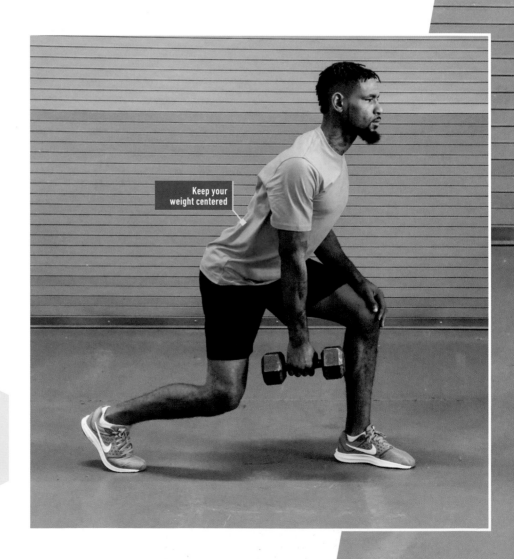

Keep your weight centered

TIP
Continually engage your core to keep your body balanced.

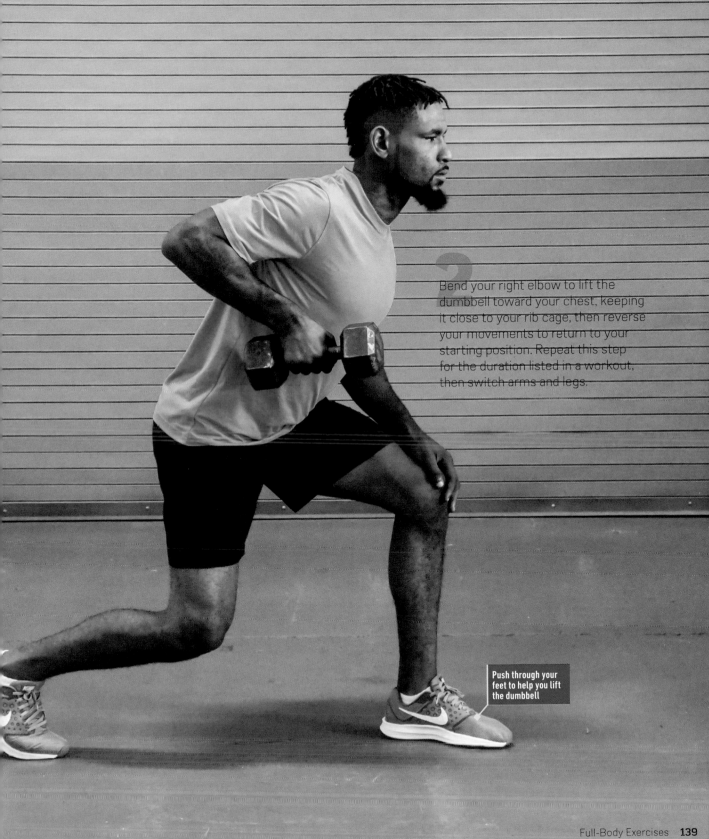

Bend your right elbow to lift the dumbbell toward your chest, keeping it close to your rib cage, then reverse your movements to return to your starting position. Repeat this step for the duration listed in a workout, then switch arms and legs.

Push through your feet to help you lift the dumbbell

STRAIGHT-LEG ROCKERS

This exercise involves two Pilates essentials: control and balance. You'll continuously engage your abs while also gaining trunk stabilization and spinal articulation. Momentum is key in gaining the flow and flexibility.

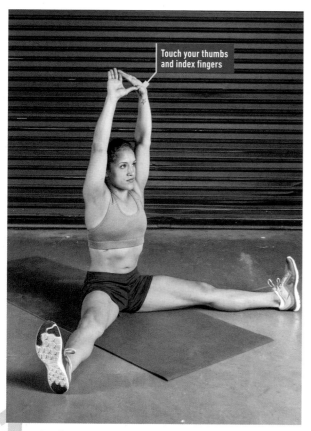

Touch your thumbs and index fingers

Sit on the floor, spreading your legs out in front of you and extending your arms above your head.

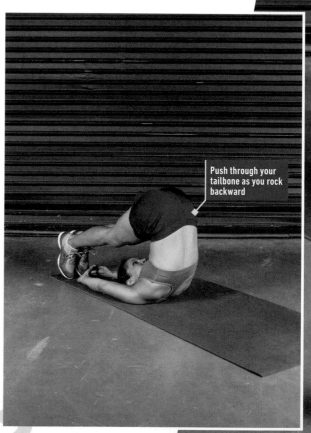

Push through your tailbone as you rock backward

Tuck your chin into your chest and rock backward, swinging your legs over your head and putting your arms flat on the ground. When your feet touch the ground, push through your toes to rock forward.

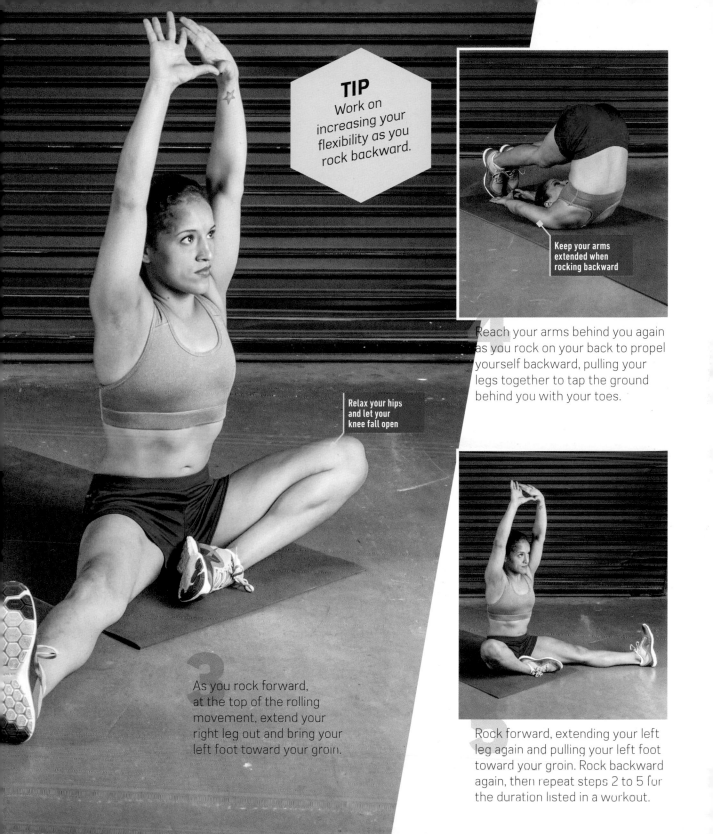

TIP
Work on increasing your flexibility as you rock backward.

Keep your arms extended when rocking backward

Reach your arms behind you again as you rock on your back to propel yourself backward, pulling your legs together to tap the ground behind you with your toes.

Relax your hips and let your knee fall open

As you rock forward, at the top of the rolling movement, extend your right leg out and bring your left foot toward your groin.

Rock forward, extending your left leg again and pulling your left foot toward your groin. Rock backward again, then repeat steps 2 to 5 for the duration listed in a workout.

SIDE SCISSORS

This exercise strengthens your abs, obliques, and lats—muscles that are key in contributing to a strong and defined core. Working one side of your body at a time can also help you develop better balance.

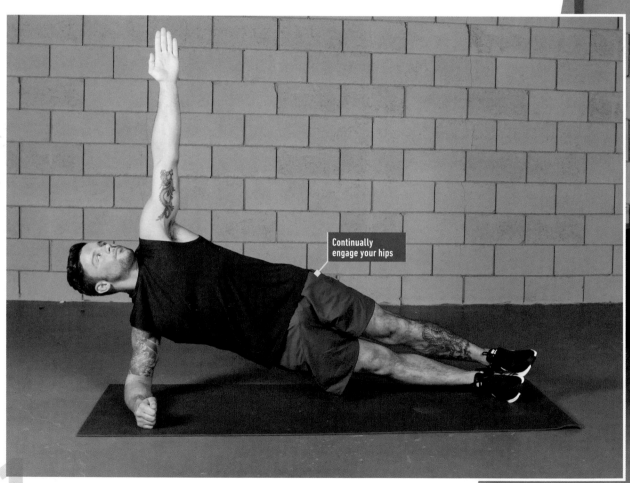

Continually engage your hips

1 Lie on your right side, stacking your feet with your right elbow and forearm on the ground and your left arm relaxed at your side. Push through your right forearm to lift your upper body off the ground, raising your hips to form a straight decline from your shoulders and extending your left arm up in the air.

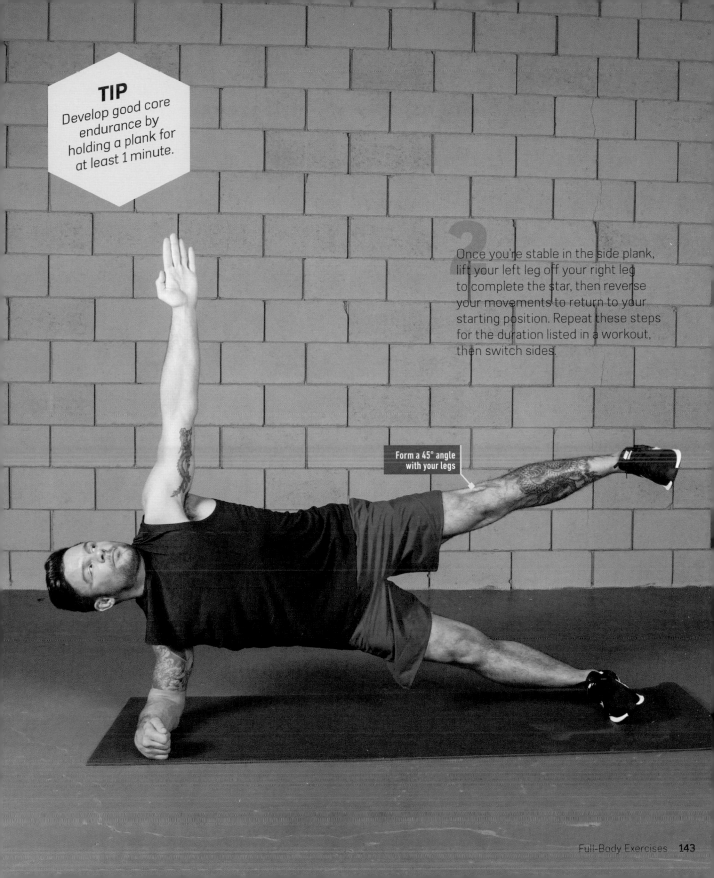

TIP
Develop good core
endurance by
holding a plank for
at least 1 minute.

2 Once you're stable in the side plank, lift your left leg off your right leg to complete the star, then reverse your movements to return to your starting position. Repeat these steps for the duration listed in a workout, then switch sides.

Form a 45° angle
with your legs

ELBOW-TO-ANKLE LUNGES

This exercise stretches and strengthens your lower body, back, hips, and shoulder muscles. Focus on technique to ensure you're strengthening and benefitting both sides of your body equally.

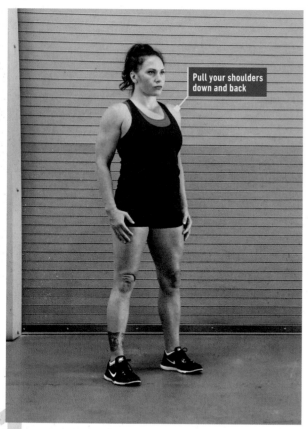

Pull your shoulders down and back

Stand with your feet hip-width apart and your arms relaxed at your sides.

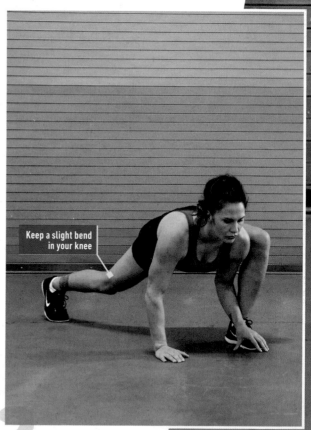

Keep a slight bend in your knee

Bend your left knee to form a 90° angle and slightly bend your right knee as you lower yourself to the ground, placing your left elbow inside your left instep.

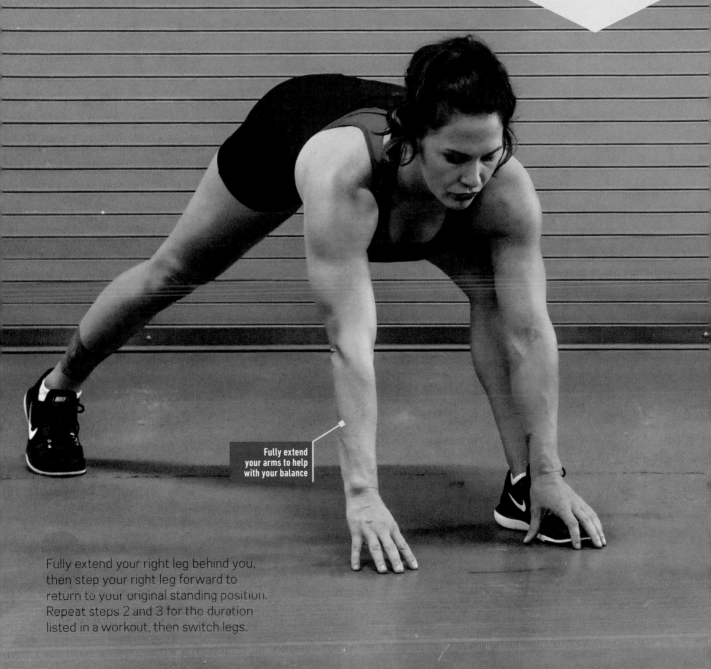

TIP
Keep moving forward rather than remaining in the same spot.

Fully extend your arms to help with your balance

Fully extend your right leg behind you, then step your right leg forward to return to your original standing position. Repeat steps 2 and 3 for the duration listed in a workout, then switch legs.

SPIDER CRAWL

Almost nothing helps you develop isometric muscles more than an exercise that demands you support your weight with your arms and legs. Continually engage your core, and work toward moving quickly and taking larger steps.

1 Put your hands flat on the ground, pointing your fingers forward, and balance your body on the flexed balls of your feet.

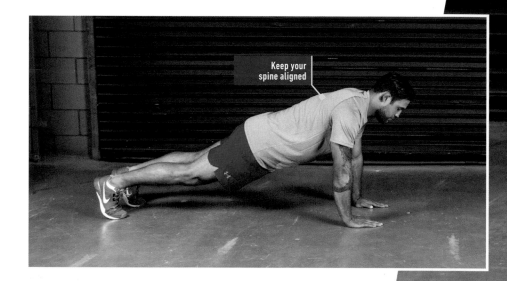

Keep your spine aligned

2 Bend your right knee to step your right foot forward to outside your right hand, keeping your right foot flat on the ground and your body balanced on the ball of your left foot.

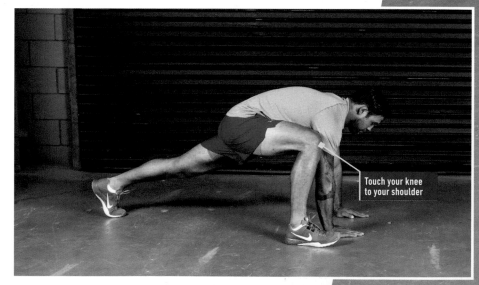

Touch your knee to your shoulder

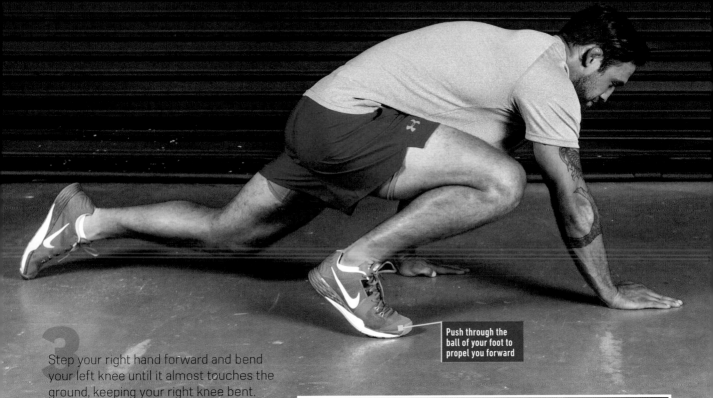

Push through the ball of your foot to propel you forward

3 Step your right hand forward and bend your left knee until it almost touches the ground, keeping your right knee bent.

4 Simultaneously walk your left hand forward to parallel with your right hand as you step your left foot forward to outside your left hand. Bend your right knee until it almost touches the ground, then step your left hand forward and bring your left knee toward your left elbow. Repeat steps 2 to 4 for the duration listed in a workout.

INCHWORM

This exercise can help you stretch and tone in multiple areas as well as increase your muscular endurance, flexibility, energy, and strength.

1 Stand with your feet hip-width apart and bend at your hips to place your hands on the ground, putting your right hand in front of your left hand.

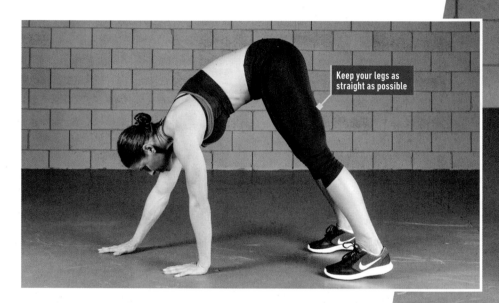

Keep your legs as straight as possible

2 Slowly walk your hands forward, alternating as you go, as you begin to lower yourself to the ground.

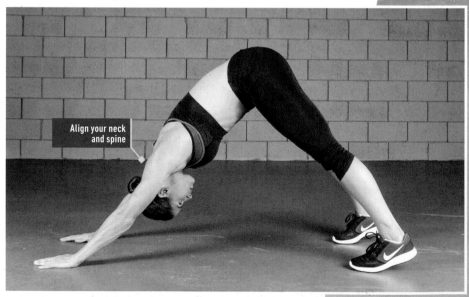

Align your neck and spine

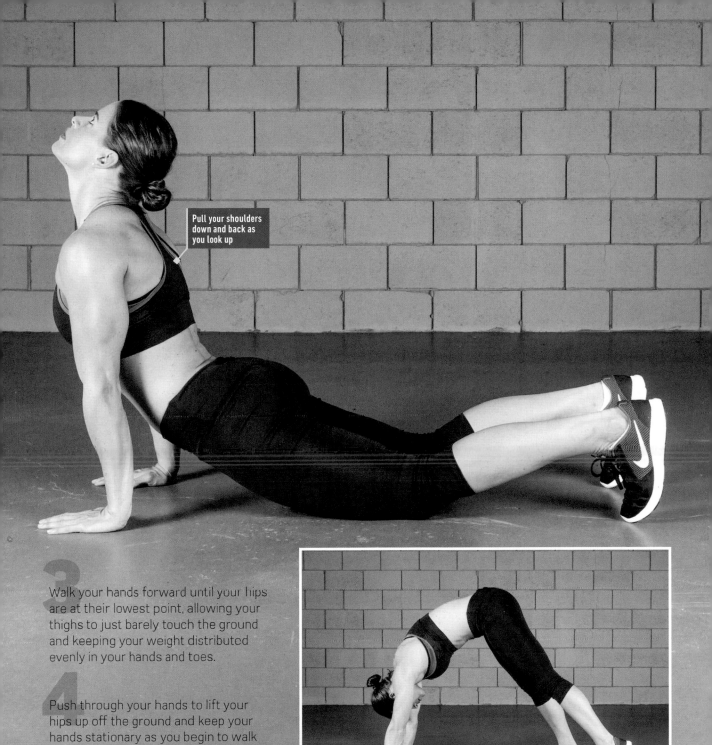

Pull your shoulders down and back as you look up

3
Walk your hands forward until your hips are at their lowest point, allowing your thighs to just barely touch the ground and keeping your weight distributed evenly in your hands and toes.

4
Push through your hands to lift your hips up off the ground and keep your hands stationary as you begin to walk your feet forward toward your hands, keeping your legs as straight as possible. Repeat steps 2 to 4 for the duration listed in a workout.

MEDICINE BALL BURPEES

You won't find many exercises as thorough as burpees. Adding a medicine ball to this classic exercise can make a stronger and more explosive impact on your entire body.

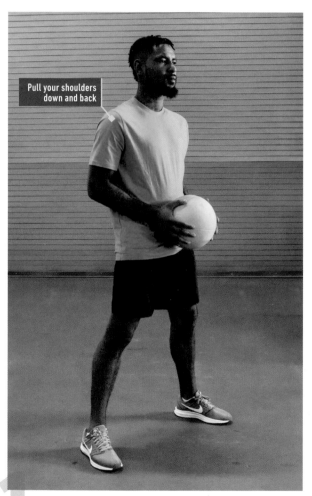

Pull your shoulders down and back

1 Stand with your feet hip-width apart, holding a medicine ball in both hands at your stomach and keeping your chin down.

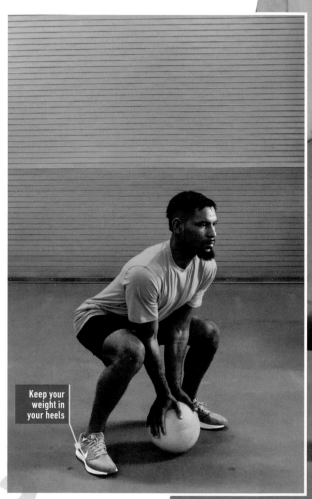

Keep your weight in your heels

2 Bend your knees to lower yourself into a squat position, shifting your hands to the top of the ball, then touch the ball to the ground.

Maintain your head, neck, and back alignment

Keep your weight in your palms and feet

Jump both feet backward, keeping them 2 feet wide and keeping your arms extended in the plank position.

Jump both feet forward to return them to their starting positions next to the ball, switching your hands to the sides of the ball, then stand to return to your starting position. Repeat steps 2 to 4 for the duration listed in a workout.

TARGETS /// shoulders, back, core, forearms, and legs
EQUIPMENT /// kettlebells

FARMER'S WALK

This exercise might seem simple, but it can strengthen and balance your motions, imperative to creating the symmetry for the body you want. This works your big muscle groups as well as tightens less obvious areas.

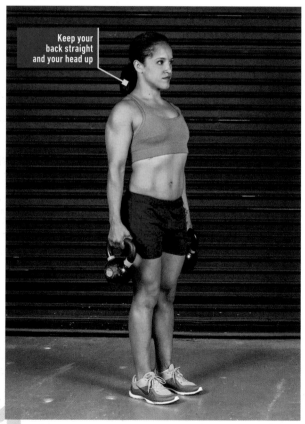

Keep your back straight and your head up

1 Stand with your feet close together and hold a kettlebell in each hand, relaxing your arms at your sides and keeping your chin down.

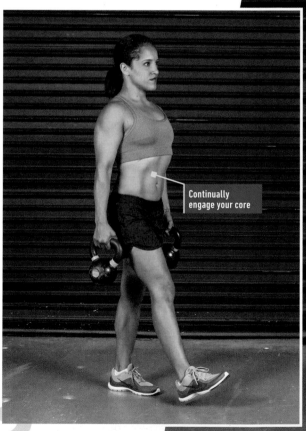

Continually engage your core

2 Step your right foot forward, touching your heel to the ground and then your toes, and keep your arms straight.

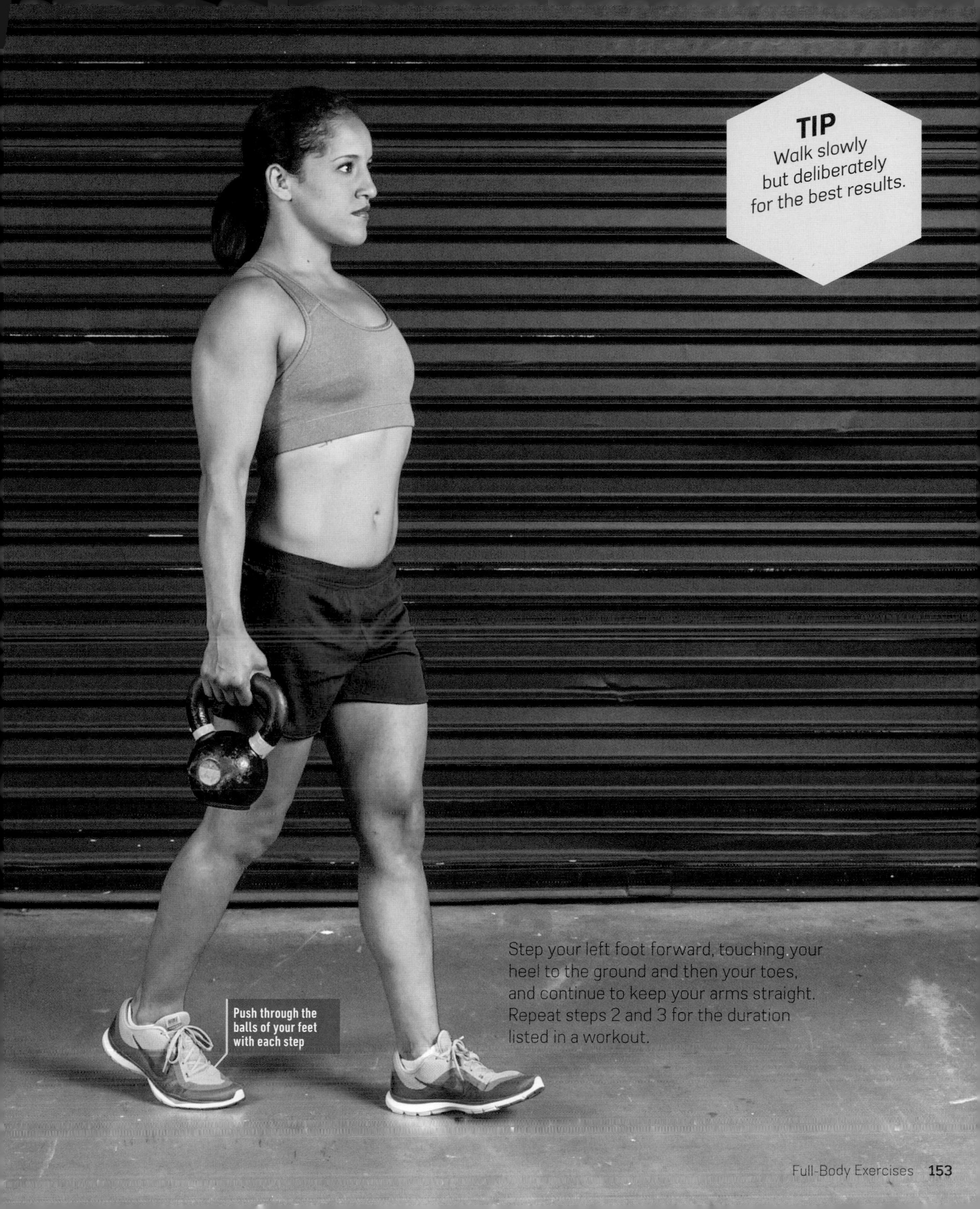

TIP
Walk slowly
but deliberately
for the best results.

Push through the
balls of your feet
with each step

Step your left foot forward, touching your
heel to the ground and then your toes,
and continue to keep your arms straight.
Repeat steps 2 and 3 for the duration
listed in a workout.

TARGETS /// abs, obliques, quads, hamstrings, glutes, triceps, trapezius, and deltoids
EQUIPMENT /// kettlebell

TURKISH SITUPS

This exercise requires you to use your whole body in cooperation with a kettlebell, helping you become more proficient with everyday movement and mobility.

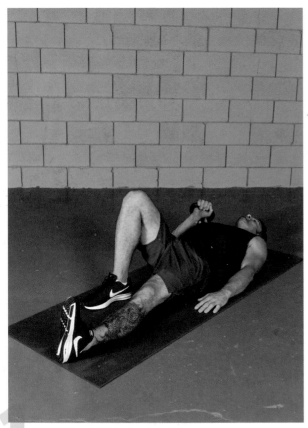

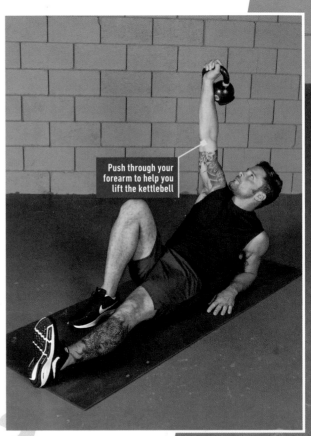

Push through your forearm to help you lift the kettlebell

Lie on your back on the floor with your legs hip-width apart and a kettlebell at your right shoulder. Bend your right knee to place your right foot flat on the ground and opposite your left knee.

Bend slightly at your hips and push up onto your left elbow as you raise your right arm, extending it straight about your right shoulder.

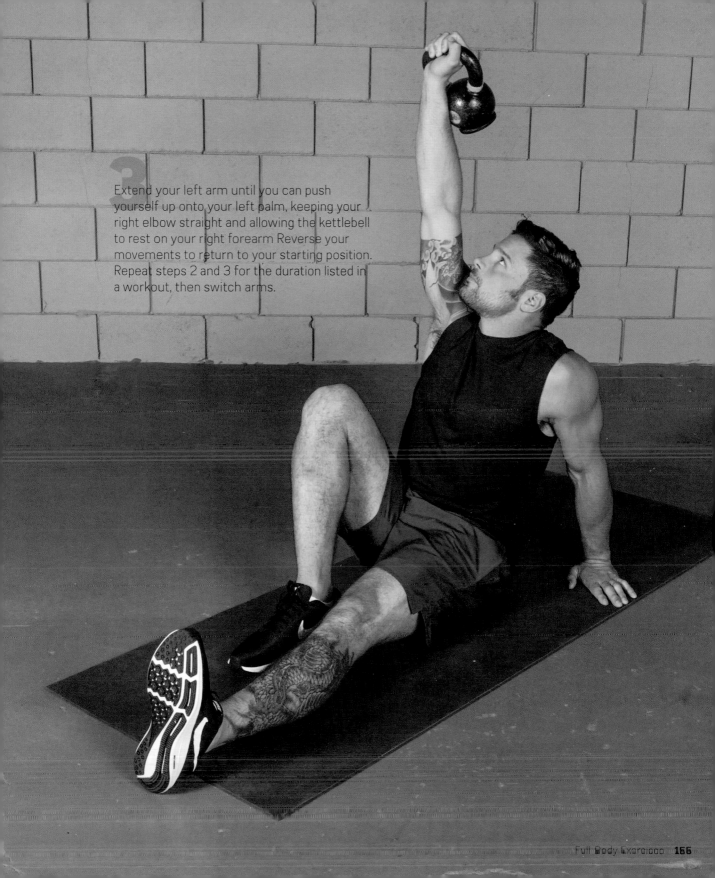

3

Extend your left arm until you can push yourself up onto your left palm, keeping your right elbow straight and allowing the kettlebell to rest on your right forearm Reverse your movements to return to your starting position. Repeat steps 2 and 3 for the duration listed in a workout, then switch arms.

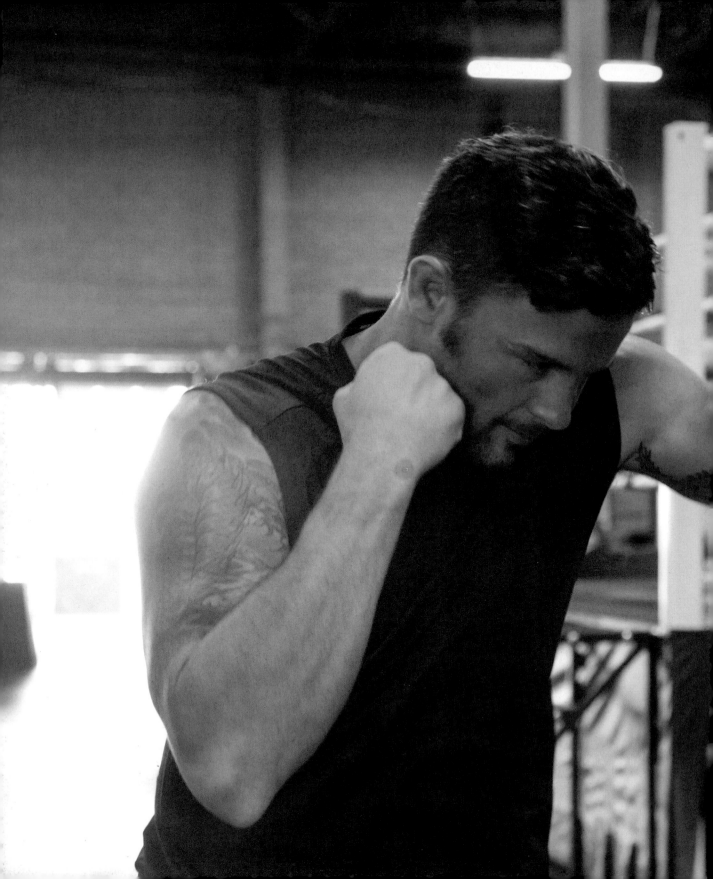

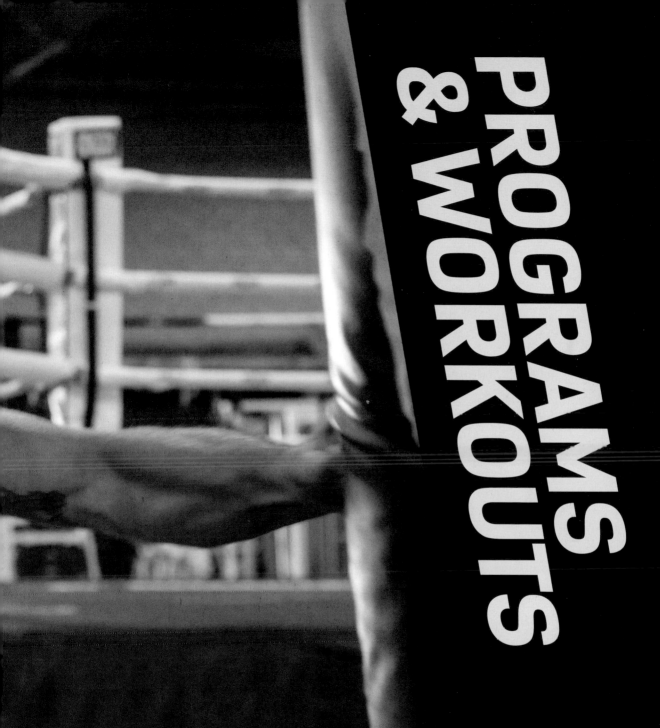

PROGRAMS & WORKOUTS

STRENGTH PROGRAM

Your physical stamina depends on how fit and how strong you are. This program helps you develop strength from top to bottom, giving you confidence to take on any challenge.

	WEEK 1	WEEK 2	WEEK 3	WEEK 4
DAY 1	Up, Down & Out p. 165	Bottoms Up p. 160	The Time Is Meow p. 162	Rest
DAY 2	Handle It p. 167	Chasing Air p. 161	Sorry, Not Sorry p. 164	Down & Dirty p. 166
DAY 3	Bottoms Up p. 160	Handle It p. 167	Rest	Up, Down & Out p. 165
DAY 4	Sorry, Not Sorry p. 164	Up, Down & Out p. 165	Down & Dirty p. 166	Sorry, Not Sorry p. 164
DAY 5	The Time Is Meow p. 162	Rest	Chasing Air p. 161	The Time Is Meow p. 162
DAY 6	Down & Dirty p. 166	Sorry, Not Sorry p. 164	Handle It p. 167	Bottoms Up p. 160
DAY 7	Rest	Down & Dirty p. 166	Bottoms Up p. 160	Handle It p. 167

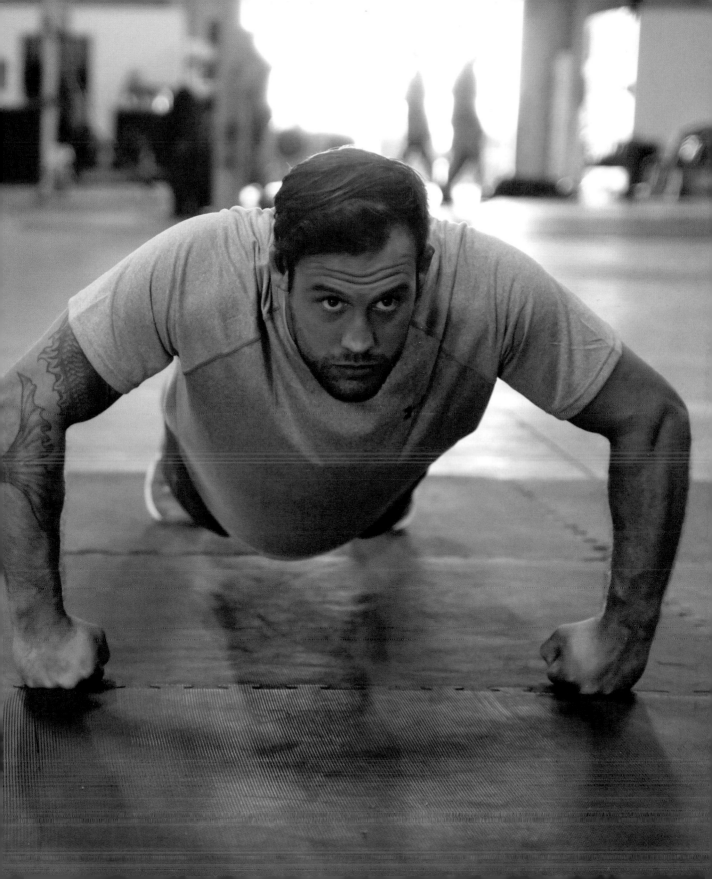

**Perform these circuits
in order three times
for an effective workout.**

EXERCISE	DURATION	PAGE
Platform step-ups	60 secs	94
Medicine ball burpees	8 reps	150
Kettlebell pulls	20 secs	70
Rest	30 secs	

EXERCISE	DURATION	PAGE
Backward lunges	10 reps per leg	102
Push kicks	6 reps per leg	86
Glute march	6 reps per side	72
Rest	30 secs	

EXERCISE	DURATION	PAGE
One-armed press	6 reps per arm	44
Elbow taps	6 reps per arm	38
Straight-leg rockers	9 reps per leg	140
Rest	30 secs	

OBJECTIVE /// to enhance muscle control
EQUIPMENT /// plyometric box, medicine ball, heavy bag, and kettlebell

BOTTOMS UP

This workout mixes familiar MMA techniques with practical but simulated motions. Starting from the legs and going up, put your mind in fight mode and smash through every set.

OBJECTIVE **///** to tone muscles
EQUIPMENT **///** medicine ball

CHASING AIR

Increase your strength and speed with these explosive and muscle-engaging motions. Yes, they're tough and demanding, but you can bend them to your will.

Perform these circuits in order three times for an effective workout.

CIRCUIT 1

EXERCISE	DURATION	PAGE
High skips	20 yards each way	126
Side scissors	45 secs	142
Overhead slams	6 reps	78
Rest	30 secs	

CIRCUIT 2

EXERCISE	DURATION	PAGE
Medicine ball punches	12 reps	30
Backward squat steps	10 reps each leg	106
Heel-to-toe rockers & squats	10 reps	110
Rest	30 secs	

CIRCUIT 3

EXERCISE	DURATION	PAGE
Medicine ball jumps	5 reps	88
Carioca	20 yards each way	64
Farmer's walk	20 yards each way	152
Rest	30 secs	

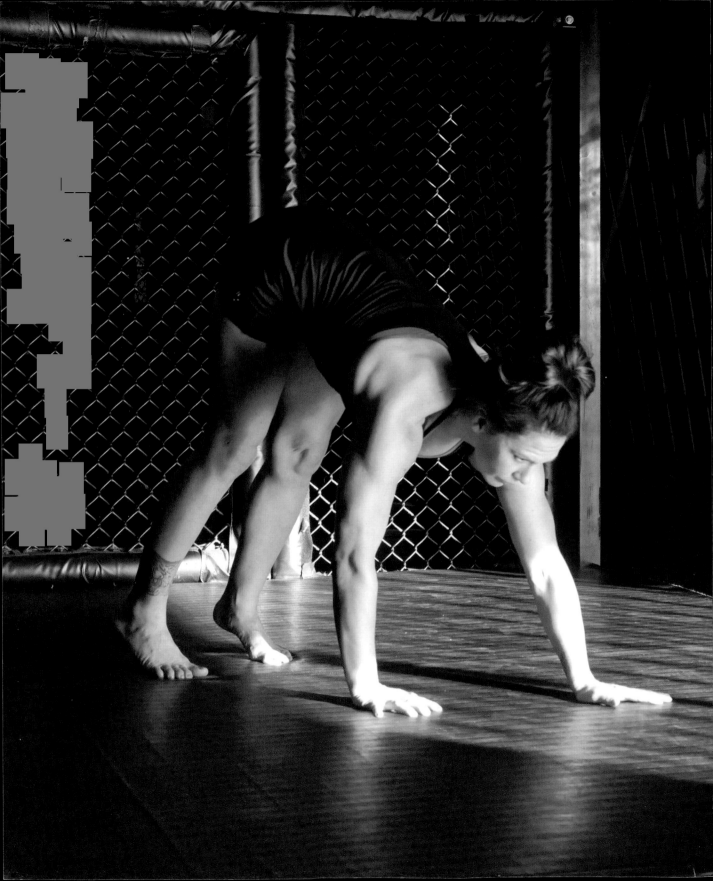

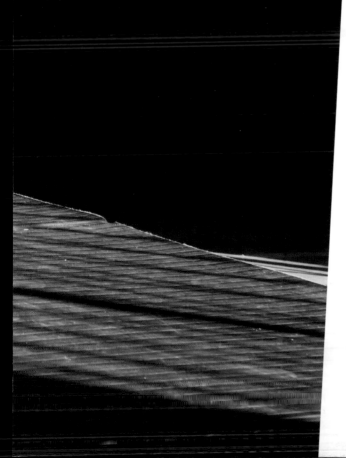

OBJECTIVE **///** **to increase overall strength**
EQUIPMENT **///** **barbell plate, step platform, and medicine ball**

THE TIME IS MEOW

Strong and dynamic legs and core can make the difference in mobility in everyday performance. No better time to make the necessary improvements than right *meow*!

Perform these circuits in order three times for an effective workout.

CIRCUIT 1	EXERCISE	DURATION	PAGE
	One-legged weight drops	6 reps	52
	Medicine ball lateral lunges	12 reps	130
	Inchworm	6 reps	148
	Rest	30 secs	

CIRCUIT 2	EXERCISE	DURATION	PAGE
	Single-hip thrusts	6 reps	114
	Carioca	20 yards each way	64
	Backward overhead throws	3 reps	82
	Rest	30 secs	

CIRCUIT 3	EXERCISE	DURATION	PAGE
	Medicine ball situps	15 secs	48
	Squat steps	10 reps	104
	Knee-to-elbow touches	12 reps	56
	Rest	30 secs	

Perform these circuits
in order three times
for an effective workout.

OBJECTIVE /// to increase strength
EQUIPMENT /// medicine ball, barbell
with weights, and plyometric box

SORRY, NOT SORRY

Who you are is perfect—
make no apology for the
madness. Meet your match in
intensity as you strengthen
from the inside out.

CIRCUIT 1

EXERCISE	DURATION	PAGE
Medicine ball squat tosses	8 reps	122
Floor press	5 reps	34
Glute march	12 reps	72
Rest	30 secs	

CIRCUIT 2

EXERCISE	DURATION	PAGE
Medicine ball burpees	6 reps	150
Heel-to-toe rockers & squats	10 reps	110
Side kicks	10 reps	92
Rest	30 secs	

CIRCUIT 3

EXERCISE	DURATION	PAGE
Platform step-ups	30 secs	94
Overhead slams	6 reps	78
Side scissors	45 secs	142
Rest	30 secs	

OBJECTIVE /// to increase kinetic energy
EQUIPMENT /// medicine ball and kettlebell

UP, DOWN & OUT

Enjoy the brief rest periods in this workout because you're going to have to change positions quickly—from up to down to out.

Perform these circuits in order three times for an effective workout.

CIRCUIT 1	EXERCISE	DURATION	PAGE
	Single-leg squats	5 reps per leg	112
	Elbow taps	6 reps per side	38
	Shadow boxing	20 secs	120
	Rest	30 secs	

CIRCUIT 2	EXERCISE	DURATION	PAGE
	Medicine ball situps	6 reps	48
	Backward lunges	20 secs	102
	Medicine ball twist	20 secs	66
	Rest	30 secs	

CIRCUIT 3	EXERCISE	DURATION	PAGE
	One-armed kettlebell carry	20 secs	50
	Squat jumps	6 reps	98
	Side scissors	45 secs	142
	Rest	30 secs	

**Perform these circuits
in order three times
for an effective workout.**

CIRCUIT 1

EXERCISE	DURATION	PAGE
Medicine ball burpees	8 reps	150
Side scissors	20 secs	142
Shadow boxing	20 secs	120
Rest	30 secs	

CIRCUIT 2

EXERCISE	DURATION	PAGE
Tempo pushups	20 reps	32
Straight-leg rockers	6 reps	140
Glute march	6 reps per leg	72
Rest	30 secs	

CIRCUIT 3

EXERCISE	DURATION	PAGE
T-shirt curls	20 secs	60
One-armed kettlebell carry	15 secs	50
Ground & pound	20 secs	128
Rest	30 secs	

OBJECTIVE /// to build confidence
EQUIPMENT /// T-shirt, kettlebell,
heavy bag, and medicine ball

DOWN & DIRTY

Challenge yourself by digging down and dirty mentally to bring your body tightness, balance, and strength to the next level.

OBJECTIVE /// to build trunk support
EQUIPMENT /// dumbbells and medicine ball

HANDLE IT

Using equipment as well as movements similar to those in fighting can help you develop that MMA body. Handling the workload with practicality in mind makes goals easily attainable.

Perform these circuits in order three times for an effective workout.

CIRCUIT 1

EXERCISE	DURATION	PAGE
Goblet carry	16 reps	132
Sit-out rotation	6 reps	134
Medicine ball chest press	6 reps	36
Rest	30 secs	

CIRCUIT 2

EXERCISE	DURATION	PAGE
Farmer's walk	20 yards each way	152
Side kicks	5 reps per side	92
Running backward	20 yards each way	100
Rest	30 secs	

CIRCUIT 3

EXERCISE	DURATION	PAGE
One-armed dumbbell row	6 reps per side	138
Bird dog	6 reps per side	62
Arm circles	20 secs each arm	40
Rest	30 secs	

STABILITY PROGRAM

You're ready to take your stability to the next level. This should be taken on its own...

	WEEK 1	WEEK 2	WEEK 3	WEEK 4
DAY 1	It Takes Balls p. 173	Foot Fire p. 171	It Takes Balls p. 173	Rest
DAY 2	Mama Said p. 170	Bad Intentions p. 172	Rock to the Beat p. 175	Legs for Daze p. 174
DAY 3	Foot Fire p. 171	Rock to the Beat p. 175	Rest	It Takes Balls p. 173
DAY 4	Rock to the Beat p. 175	It Takes Balls p. 173	Mama Said p. 170	Bad Intentions p. 172
DAY 5	Bad Intentions p. 172	Rest	Foot Fire p. 171	Rock to the Beat p. 175
DAY 6	Legs for Daze p. 174	Mama Said p. 170	Legs for Daze p. 174	Mama Said p. 170
DAY 7	Rest	Legs for Daze p. 174	Bad Intentions p. 172	Foot Fire p. 171

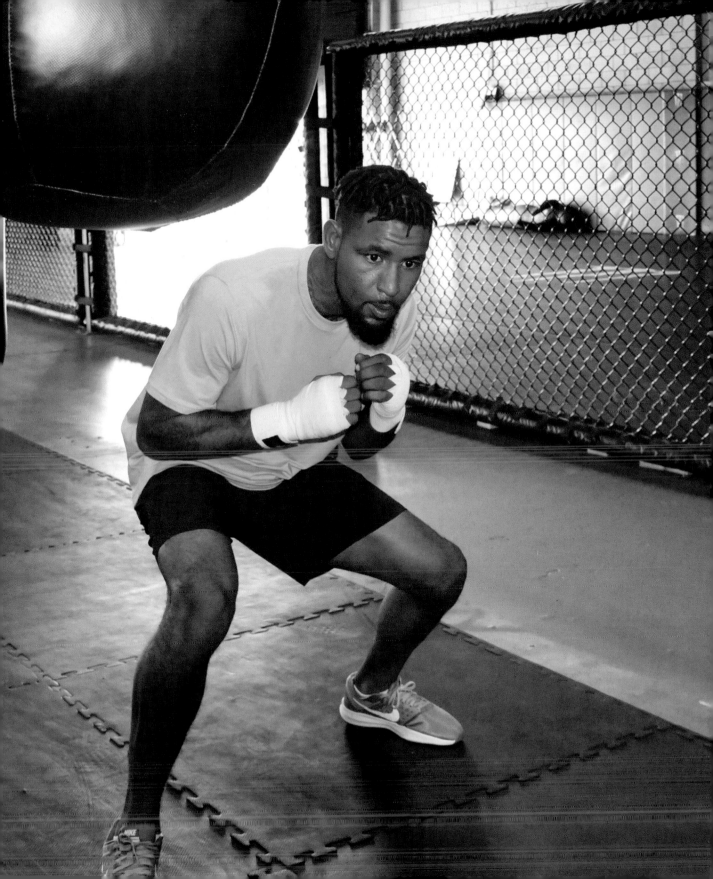

**Perform these circuits
in order three times
for an effective workout.**

OBJECTIVE /// to regain control
EQUIPMENT /// speed bag, heavy bag,
medicine ball, and kettlebell

MAMA SAID

She said there'd be days like this, and getting through them is the prize. Push yourself until you make Mama proud, then stand tall because you did it!

CIRCUIT 1

EXERCISE	DURATION	PAGE
Medicine ball wall sit	20 secs	380
Running backward	20 yards each way	100
Ground & pound	20 secs	128
Rest	30 secs	

CIRCUIT 2

EXERCISE	DURATION	PAGE
Medicine ball lateral lunges	6 reps per leg	130
Inchworm	6 reps	148
Pushup rotation	3 reps per side	136
Rest	30 secs	

CIRCUIT 3

EXERCISE	DURATION	PAGE
Medicine ball hip throws	3 reps per arm	76
Squat steps	15 secs per leg	104
Turkish situps	8 reps	154
Rest	30 secs	

OBJECTIVE *///* to increase stability
EQUIPMENT *///* soccer ball

FOOT FIRE

Your endurance depends on your legs more than any other body part, and this workout sets you aflame with enhancing and strengthening your power, agility, and lasting performance. Make sure you shake out between each continuous set.

Perform these circuits in order three times for an effective workout.

CIRCUIT 1

EXERCISE	DURATION	PAGE
Farmer's walk	20 secs each way	152
Soccer ball touches	15 reps	116
Side scissors	45 secs	142
Rest	30 secs	

CIRCUIT 2

EXERCISE	DURATION	PAGE
Sit-out rotation	6 reps	134
Side-to-side shuffle	15 secs	90
Backward squat steps	10 reps	106
Rest	30 secs	

CIRCUIT 3

EXERCISE	DURATION	PAGE
Plank drop to elbows	12 reps	58
Side kicks	5 reps per leg	92
Heel-to-toe rockers & squats	10 reps	110
Rest	30 secs	

**Perform these circuits
in order three times
for an effective workout.**

EXERCISE	DURATION	PAGE
Box jumps	5 reps	68
Overhead slams	5 reps	78
Bird dog	8 reps	62
Rest	30 secs	

EXERCISE	DURATION	PAGE
Kettlebell punches	30 secs	42
Carioca	20 yards each way	64
Inchworm	30 secs	148
Rest	30 secs	

EXERCISE	DURATION	PAGE
Medicine ball squats	8 reps	96
Floor press	5 reps	34
Lateral crawl	15 secs per side	124
Rest	30 secs	

OBJECTIVE **///** to develop agility
EQUIPMENT **///** plyometric box, medicine ball, kettlebell, and barbell with weights

BAD INTENTIONS

Be victorious no matter what. These dynamic motions use and encourage results in every part of your body. No matter the intention, take personal accountability in completing this workout with success.

OBJECTIVE **///** to increase dexterity
EQUIPMENT **///** medicine ball, dumbbells,
and soccer ball

IT TAKES BALLS

Adding weight or resistance creates accountability in form and commitment to improving workout habits. Measure your growth and endurance while you push yourself time and time again.

Perform these circuits in order three times for an effective workout.

CIRCUIT 1

EXERCISE	DURATION	PAGE
Medicine ball hip throws	10 reps per side	76
Lateral crawl	15 secs per side	124
Medicine ball twist	17 reps per side	66
Rest	30 secs	

CIRCUIT 2

EXERCISE	DURATION	PAGE
One-armed dumbbell row	6 reps per side	138
Medicine ball chest press	6 reps	36
Soccer ball touches	30 secs	116
Rest	30 secs	

CIRCUIT 3

EXERCISE	DURATION	PAGE
One-legged weight drops	6 reps	52
Goblet carry	16 reps per leg	132
Side scissors	45 secs	142
Rest	30 secs	

Perform these circuits
in order three times
for an effective workout.

EXERCISE	DURATION	PAGE
Running backward	20 yards each way	100
Sit-out rotation	6 reps	134
Medicine ball squats	5 reps	96
Rest	60 secs	

EXERCISE	DURATION	PAGE
Medicine ball jumps	5 reps	88
Carioca	20 yards each way	64
Backward squat steps	10 reps	106
Rest	30 secs	

EXERCISE	DURATION	PAGE
Medicine ball hip throws	6 reps	76
Single-hip thrusts	6 reps	114
T-shirt curls	20 secs per side	60
Rest	30 secs	

OBJECTIVE /// to fortify balance
EQUIPMENT /// medicine ball, step platform, and T-shirt

LEGS FOR DAZE

Having strong legs when the going gets tough can give you the advantage you need to persevere. Push through these now and thank yourself later.

OBJECTIVE /// to improve balance
EQUIPMENT /// soccer ball, medicine ball, step platform, and plyometric box

ROCK TO THE BEAT

Find your rhythm during this workout, but continually remain focused on form to ensure you get the most from these diverse and technical exercises.

Perform these circuits in order three times for an effective workout.

CIRCUIT 1

EXERCISE	DURATION	PAGE
Platform step-ups	45 secs	94
Knee-to-elbow touches	12 reps	56
Sit-out rotation	6 reps	134
Rest	30 secs	

CIRCUIT 2

EXERCISE	DURATION	PAGE
Soccer ball touches	30 secs	116
Squat steps	10 reps	104
Side scissors	10 reps	142
Rest	30 secs	

CIRCUIT 3

EXERCISE	DURATION	PAGE
Medicine ball lateral lunges	12 reps	130
Pushup rotation	6 reps	136
Bird dog	12 reps	62
Rest	30 secs	

POWER PROGRAM

If you're looking for more force and more speed in your everyday life, increasing your muscle command can help. This program boosts your power and renews your focus on form.

	WEEK 1	WEEK 2	WEEK 3	WEEK 4
DAY 1	Cat Be Nimble p. 180	Can't Touch This p. 183	Get Down, Get Down p. 178	Rest
DAY 2	Get Your Mind Right p. 184	Overtaker p. 179	Can't Touch This p. 183	Cat Be Nimble p. 180
DAY 3	Overtaker p. 179	Get Down, Get Down p. 178	Rest	Can't Touch This p. 183
DAY 4	Get Down, Get Down p. 178	Get Off Me p. 182	Overtaker p. 179	Get Your Mind Right p. 184
DAY 5	Leave It All Out There p. 186	Rest	Cat Be Nimble p. 180	Get Off Me p. 182
DAY 6	Get Off Me p. 182	Get Your Mind Right p. 184	Get Off Me p. 182	Get Down, Get Down p. 178
DAY 7	Rest	Cat Be Nimble p. 180	Get Your Mind Right p. 184	Leave It All Out There p. 186

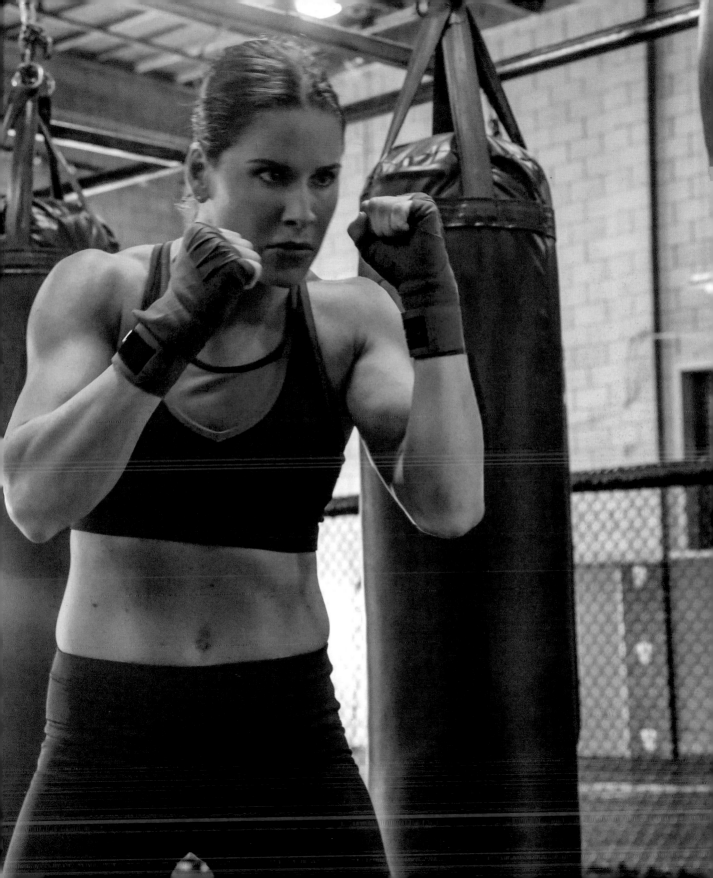

**Perform these circuits
in order three times
for an effective workout.**

CIRCUIT 1

EXERCISE	DURATION	PAGE
Backward overhead throws	5 reps	82
Side scissors	45 secs	142
Spider crawl	30 secs	146
Rest	90 secs	

CIRCUIT 2

EXERCISE	DURATION	PAGE
Arm circles	20 reps each way	40
Tempo pushups	30 secs	32
Shadow boxing	30 secs	120
Rest	90 secs	

CIRCUIT 3

EXERCISE	DURATION	PAGE
Medicine ball twist	17 reps per side	66
Lateral crawl	15 secs each way	124
Ground & pound	20 secs	128
Rest	90 secs	

OBJECTIVE /// to strengthen pace
EQUIPMENT /// medicine ball

GET DOWN, GET DOWN

You'll definitely get down—on the ground and with repeated motions—as you find and develop your rhythm to each exercise's movements.

OBJECTIVE /// to increase speed
EQUIPMENT /// medicine ball, plyometric box, and kettlebell

OVERTAKER

Keep your pace even but strong during these exercises so you aren't overwhelmed—or even overtaken by their demands.

Perform these circuits in order three times for an effective workout.

CIRCUIT 1

EXERCISE	DURATION	PAGE
Medicine ball hip throws	10 reps per side	76
Box jumps	5 reps	68
Elbow-to-ankle lunges	20 secs	144
Rest	30 secs	

CIRCUIT 2

EXERCISE	DURATION	PAGE
Single-leg squats	6 reps per leg	112
Side scissors	20 secs per side	142
Straight-leg rockers	9 reps per leg	140
Rest	30 secs	

CIRCUIT 3

EXERCISE	DURATION	PAGE
Kettlebell pulls	20 secs	70
Side-to side shuffle	20 yards each way	90
Bird dog	8 reps	62
Rest	30 secs	

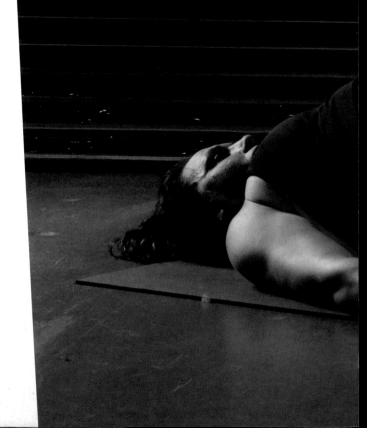

Perform these circuits
in order three times
for an effective workout.

CIRCUIT 1

EXERCISE	DURATION	PAGE
One-armed dumbbell row	6 reps	138
Squat jumps	6 reps	98
Single-armed kettlebell carry	8 reps	50
Rest	90 secs	

CIRCUIT 2

EXERCISE	DURATION	PAGE
Handstand pushups	8 reps	74
Overhead slams	6 reps	78
Jumping knees	4 reps per side	108
Rest	90 secs	

CIRCUIT 3

EXERCISE	DURATION	PAGE
Elbow taps	12 reps	38
Glute march	12 reps	72
Kettlebell punches	20 secs	42
Rest	90 secs	

OBJECTIVE /// to develop fluidity
EQUIPMENT /// dumbbells, kettlebell, and medicine ball

CAT BE NIMBLE

Be Cat-like quick with how fast you move from exercise to exercise in each circuit in this workout—a great push for your mind and body.

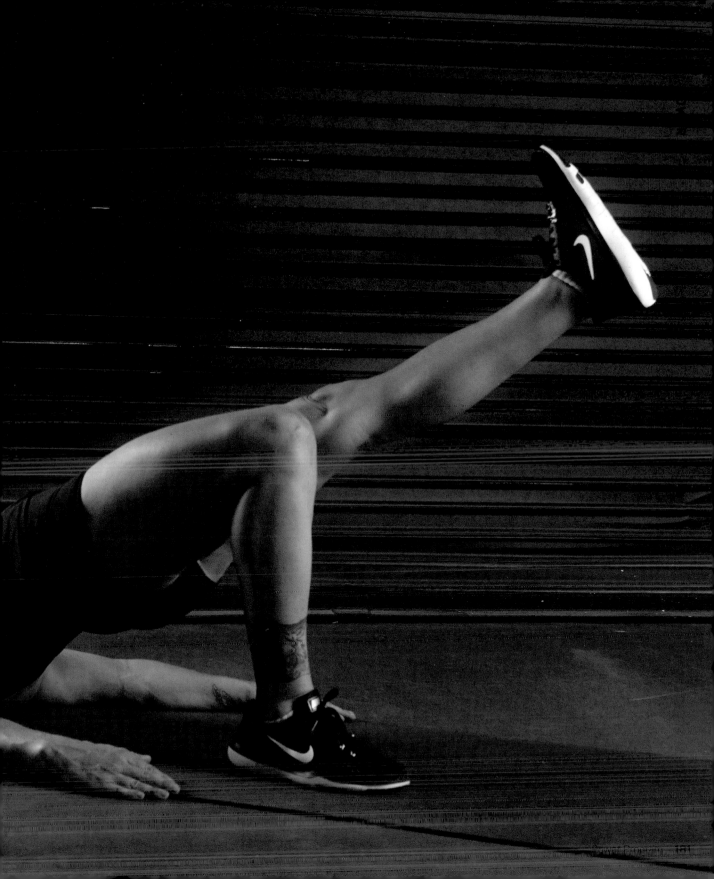

Perform these circuits in order three times for an effective workout.

GET OFF ME

This workout is definitely tough—but you're tougher. Everything in these circuits is designed to be diverse but demanding to show yourself what you're made of. You can do anything!

CIRCUIT 1

EXERCISE	DURATION	PAGE
Lateral crawl	15 secs a side	124
Medicine ball chest press	6 reps	36
Push kicks	5 reps per side	86
Rest	30 secs	

CIRCUIT 2

EXERCISE	DURATION	PAGE
Medicine ball twist	17 reps per side	66
Shadow boxing	20 secs	120
Rest	30 secs	

CIRCUIT 3

EXERCISE	DURATION	PAGE
Plank drop to elbows	20 secs	58
Inchworm	6 reps	148
High skips	20 yards each way	126
Rest	30 secs	

OBJECTIVE /// to increase concentration
EQUIPMENT /// medicine ball, heavy bag, and step platform

CAN'T TOUCH THIS

Everything involved in this workout is related to defense and offense in reaching your goals. Being agile and aggressive in intention can build confidence in your movements.

Perform these circuits in order three times for an effective workout.

CIRCUIT 1

EXERCISE	DURATION	PAGE
Push kicks	10 reps	86
Single-hip thrusts	6 reps	114
Pushup rotation	5 reps per side	136
Rest	30 secs	

CIRCUIT 2

EXERCISE	DURATION	PAGE
Jumping knees	6 reps	108
Medicine ball hip throws	6 reps per side	76
Squat steps	10 reps	104
Rest	30 secs	

CIRCUIT 3

EXERCISE	DURATION	PAGE
Arm circles	20 reps each way	40
High skips	20 yards each way	126
Ground & pound	20 secs	128
Rest	30 secs	

**Perform these circuits
in order three times
for an effective workout.**

CIRCUIT 1

EXERCISE	DURATION	PAGE
Turkish situps	6 reps	154
Shadow boxing	20 secs	120
Heel-to-toe rockers & squats	10 reps	110
Rest	30 secs	

CIRCUIT 2

EXERCISE	DURATION	PAGE
Medicine ball situps	6 reps	48
Side-to-side shuffle	20 yards each way	90
Push kicks	5 reps per side	86
Rest	30 secs	

CIRCUIT 3

EXERCISE	DURATION	PAGE
Medicine ball hip throws	6 per side	76
Box jumps	5 reps	68
Plank drop to elbows	20 secs	58
Rest	30 secs	

OBJECTIVE **///** to increase repetition
EQUIPMENT **///** kettlebell, medicine ball,
heavy bag, and plyometric box

GET YOUR MIND RIGHT

Every time you push beyond
your comfort zone, you define
the new level of your limits.
Be resilient in this workout
and keep your mind right for
your goals.

OBJECTIVE /// to enhance range of motion
EQUIPMENT /// heavy bag, medicine ball,
and step platform

LEAVE IT ALL OUT THERE

Finishing stronger than you started is how you'll go from ordinary to extraordinary. Walk away from training knowing you did your best, and remember to benchmark your progress.

Perform these circuits in order three times for an effective workout.

CIRCUIT 1

EXERCISE	DURATION	PAGE
Push kicks	10 reps	86
Medicine ball burpees	8 reps	150
Side-to-side shuffle	20 yards each way	90
Rest	30 secs	

CIRCUIT 2

EXERCISE	DURATION	PAGE
One-armed press	6 reps per side	44
Single-hip thrusts	6 reps per side	114
Shadow boxing	30 secs	120
Rest	30 secs	

CIRCUIT 3

EXERCISE	DURATION	PAGE
Backward squat steps	10 reps	106
Medicine ball twist	17 reps per side	66
Ground & pound	20 secs	128
Rest	30 secs	

INDEX

*I dedicate this book to my son, Brayden Zingano,
the young man who will forever remain my baby.
In so many ways, at different points in our lives,
Brayden has given me the drive, strength, and motivation
to keep moving forward through any and all of life's challenges.*

ABOUT THE AUTHOR

Cat Zingano is a top contending UFC fighter who held world championship belts in the Ring of Fire and Fight to Win in the bantamweight and flyweight divisions. She was also the undefeated flyweight world champion before she moved up to bantamweight. Cat's currently a world champion in Brazilian jiu-jitsu, holding a purple belt in that sport, and as a wrestler in college, she was a two-time all-American and a two-time national champion. She has wins over two UFC bantamweight champions (Miesha Tate and Amanda Nunez) and has fought in nothing but #1 contender or title fights in the last 7 years. Cat lives in San Diego with her son.

ACKNOWLEDGMENTS

I want to thank Loren Landow, Josh Ford, and all my teammates, coaches, family, friends, and students who have contributed to my success along the way. Special thanks to my other teammates—editor Christopher Stolle, designer William Thomas; art director Nigel Wright; photographer Robert Randall; and models Danyelle Wolf, Paulina Granados, Darrion Caldwell, Nick Piedmont, and Tarsis Humphreys, the models—for their help in making my dream of writing a book come true.

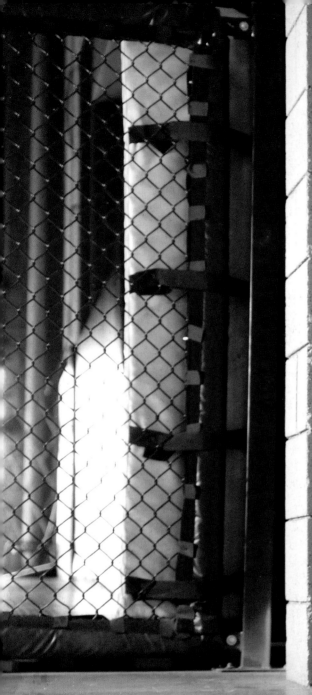

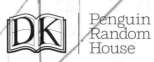

Publisher Mike Sanders
Associate publisher Billy Fields
Acquisitions editor Christopher Stolle
Development editor Christopher Stolle
Book designer William Thomas
Photographer Robert Randall
Art director Nigel Wright
Prepress technician Brian Massey
Proofreader Laura Caddell
Indexer Heather McNeill

First American Edition, 2018
Published in the United States by DK Publishing
6081 E. 82nd Street, Indianapolis, Indiana 46250

Copyright © 2018 Dorling Kindersley Limited
A Penguin Random House Company
17 18 19 20   10 9 8 7 6 5 4 3 2 1
001–308493–March/2018

Published in the United States by Dorling Kindersley Limited.

ISBN: 978-1-4654-6996-0
Library of Congress Catalog Number: 2017952281

Note: This publication contains the opinions and ideas of its author(s).
It is intended to provide helpful and informative material on the subject
matter covered. It is sold with the understanding that the author(s) and
publisher are not engaged in rendering professional services in the
book. If the reader requires personal assistance or advice, a competent
professional should be consulted. The author(s) and publisher
specifically disclaim any responsibility for any liability, loss, or risk,
personal or otherwise, which is incurred as a consequence, directly or
indirectly, of the use and application of any of the contents of this book.

Trademarks: All terms mentioned in this book that are known to be or
are suspected of being trademarks or service marks have been
appropriately capitalized. Alpha Books, DK, and Penguin Random House
LLC cannot attest to the accuracy of this information. Use of a term in
this book should not be regarded as affecting the validity of any
trademark or service mark.

DK books are available at special discounts when purchased in bulk for
sales promotions, premiums, fund-raising, or educational use. For
details, contact: DK Publishing Special Markets, 345 Hudson Street,
New York, New York 10014 or SpecialSales@dk.com.

Printed and bound in China

All images © Dorling Kindersley Limited
For further information see: www.dkimages.com

A WORLD OF IDEAS:
SEE ALL THERE IS TO KNOW
www.dk.com